United They Stand

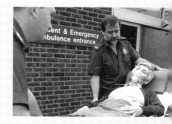

1 **Admission**

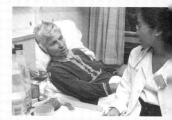

2 **Treatment**

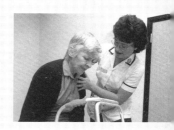

3 **Rehabilitation and the Return Home**

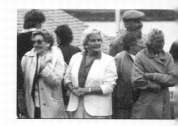

4 **Wider Lessons**

Contents

Typeset by Dominic Shearn, IDP, Bath
Printed in the UK for the Audit
Commission by Bourne Press Limited,
Bournemouth, Dorset
ISBN 011 886 434 3

London: HMSO

Photographs by Hilary Shedel and with thanks to
the staff of West Middlesex University Hospital
NHS Trust, Isleworth

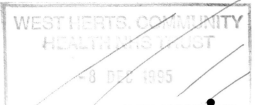

united they stand

Co-ordinating Care for Elderly Patients with Hip Fracture

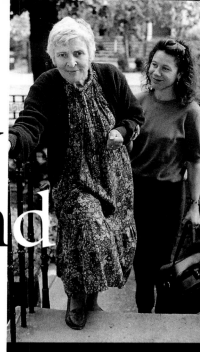

executive briefing

November 1995

The number of people who fracture their hips is rising...

- there are 57,000 each year, about one a day per hospital
- this number could double by 2015
- modern treatment improves outcomes significantly, but hospital care alone already costs over £250 million per year

...and their care needs to be well-planned and co-ordinated.

- elderly people's needs are often complex
- a wide range of hospital services is involved
- care often needs to continue after discharge

Effective care is needed right from the start...

- some people have to wait too long in casualty
- their assessment is not always sufficiently comprehensive

...and should continue throughout people's stay in hospital.

- waiting more than 24 hours for an operation is not uncommon
- operations are sometimes performed by unsupervised junior doctors
- co-ordination between surgeons and physicians specialising in elderly care medicine is sometimes poor

Few hospitals organise rehabilitation well...

- good teamwork is essential
- effective assessment and planning assist a speedier recovery
- suitable hospital environments help people to recover their confidence and independence

...or adopt a systematic approach to successful discharge.

- people needing continuing help must be identified early
- social services should be brought in early if needed

Good co-ordination of care can improve outcomes...

- strong links between physicians and surgeons can help people recover more quickly
- one person co-ordinating arrangements can ensure that the care needed is in place at each stage

...and there are wider lessons to be drawn.

- purchasers need to specify good practice
- these principles can be applied to elderly people with other conditions
- patients, relatives and carers should be kept involved and informed throughout.

A·U·D·I·T
COMMISSION

'Effective co-ordination is required if care is to be successful'

introduction

1. The number of people who fracture their hip is rising, because both the population of elderly people and the *rate* of fracture are increasing. Estimates of numbers expected in 20 years time vary between 60,000 and 117,000 hip fractures a year. Latest available figures suggest a continuing rate of growth between these two estimates (Exhibit 1).

2. If trusts are to cope, they must adopt best practices to improve recovery and maximise the number of patients who can return home – which varies significantly between hospitals (Exhibit 2). Considerable progress has been made in recent years in the treatment of hip fractures, and almost all can now be repaired surgically. Most patients can walk again within a day or two and be home in a few weeks, unless frailty or medical complications cause delay.

3. But the process of care is often complex and effective co-ordination of services is required if it is to be successful. Most patients:
- are admitted to hospital via the accident and emergency department;
- are then transferred to an orthopaedic ward for their operation;
- receive treatment for any medical conditions, often from a physician specialising in elderly care medicine;
- undergo rehabilitation by nurses and therapists after their operation; and
- return home, or move on to permanent residential or nursing home care for the first time.

Inadequate care at any stage or in the co-ordination of the whole process can lead to poorer outcomes.

Exhibit 1
Incidence of hip fracture in England and Wales

Latest available figures suggest a continuing rate of growth.

Source: Royal College of Physicians (Ref. 1) Table 4

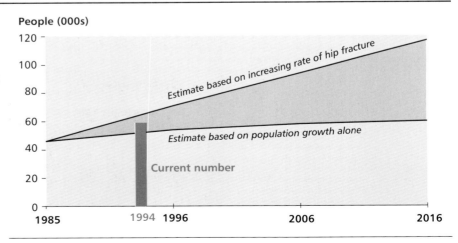

admission

'Most patients are admitted through A&E and need a full assessment of their medical, nursing and social problems'

Exhibit 2
Discharge destinations of patients admitted from home

The numbers from home who return directly home varies widely between hospitals.

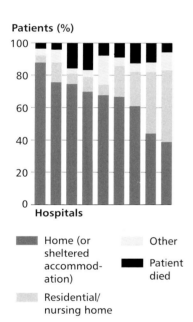

Patients (%)

Hospitals

- ■ Home (or sheltered accommodation)
- ▒ Residential/ nursing home
- ░ Other
- ■ Patient died

Source: 450 patient records from nine hospitsls

Accident and emergency

4. Almost all patients who have fractured their hips are admitted through accident and emergency (A&E) departments. Guidelines issued by the Royal College of Physicians recommend that patients wait no more than one hour in A&E (Ref. 1), but most patients wait longer (Exhibit 3).

5. There are several points where delays can occur, and some hospitals are introducing special arrangements to speed patients through. Where delays are inevitable, extra care should be taken to address the special needs of elderly people.

On to the ward

6. Because of their complex needs, hip fracture patients require a full assessment of their medical, nursing and social problems. This assessment, started in A&E, must be completed once they reach the ward and forms the basis for planning treatment and care. An incomplete assessment may fail to identify problems which subsequently cause difficulties either immediately in preparation for surgery, or in the longer term during rehabilitation and the preparation for the return home.

7. Nursing assessment, in particular, needs to be reviewed to make sure it routinely covers such key items as:

- ◆ pressure sore risk
- ◆ hydration and nutrition
- ◆ pain
- ◆ continence
- ◆ mental state
- ◆ previous mobility
- ◆ functional ability
- ◆ social circumstances

Assessments should be properly documented.

Exhibit 3
Length of time patients spend in A&E

Most patients wait longer than one hour.

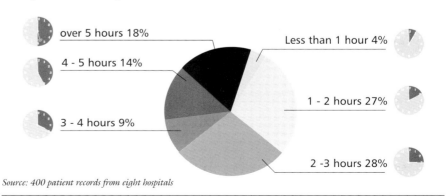

over 5 hours 18%

4 - 5 hours 14%

3 - 4 hours 9%

Less than 1 hour 4%

1 - 2 hours 27%

2 -3 hours 28%

Source: 400 patient records from eight hospitals

'Treatment involves both surgical and medical care'

treatment

Surgical care

8. More than 95 per cent of hip fracture patients have operations to repair their fracture. Although common, these operations require technical skill and experience. In the hospitals visited by the Commission there was a wide variation in the grade of surgeons and anaesthetists involved. In some hospitals, between a quarter and a half of the operations were performed by unsupervised junior orthopaedic surgeons (senior house officers, or SHOs). In others, none of the operations was unsupervised. A similar range was observed for anaesthetists, and in 10 per cent of operations both the orthopaedic doctors and anaesthetists were SHOs. While some SHOs in either specialty may have sufficient experience to work unaided on these cases, this practice should be monitored and justified.

9. Where hip fracture patients are medically fit, they should have their operations as soon as possible – preferably within 24 hours of admission (Ref. 1). This requires operating lists specifically for trauma cases, but in spite of a long-standing recommendation from the British Orthopaedic Association (Ref. 2), not all hospitals have them. As a result, patients wait longer in some hospitals than in others (Exhibit 4). Some have their operations cancelled at short notice and as a result may be 'starved for theatre' more than once. Reducing unnecessary waits for surgery both benefits patients and releases resources – an average of one or two bed-days per patient.

Medical care

10. Many patients suffer from medical conditions in addition to their fracture. Indeed, these

Exhibit 4
Waits for surgery

Patients wait longer in some hospitals than others.

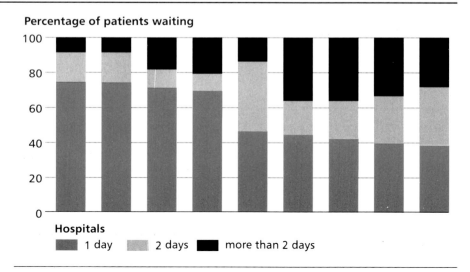

Percentage of patients waiting

Hospitals
■ 1 day ■ 2 days ■ more than 2 days

Source: 450 patient records at nine hospitals

conditions may have caused the fall and fracture in the first place. Some patients have complex social problems. As a result, many could benefit from the skills of physicians (and their teams) who specialise in elderly care medicine.

11. Arrangements to involve physicians vary widely between hospitals. Some have few formal links between orthopaedic surgeons and physicians, some have named contacts, while in others surgeons and physicians work closely together. In the Edinburgh Royal Infirmary, assessments of all new patients with hip fractures are undertaken by physicians before surgery – allowing care to be planned from the start.

12. There is some evidence (Ref. 3) that patients recover more quickly and are more likely to return to their homes when there is a close working relationship between surgeons and physicians – known as 'orthogeriatric liaison'. This is supported by findings in this study (Exhibit 5).

Exhibit 5
Effects of orthogeriatric liaison

Patients on wards with formal liaison are likely to be transferred more quickly...

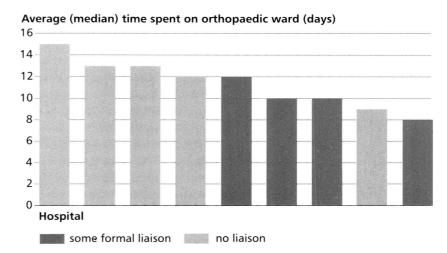

Average (median) time spent on orthopaedic ward (days)

Hospital

■ some formal liaison   ▨ no liaison

...and are more likely to return home.

Proportion of patients admitted from home who go directly home

Hospital

■ some formal liaison   ▨ no liaison

Source: 450 patient records at nine hospitals

'Efficient rehabilitation requires good teamwork and effective planning'

rehabilitation

13. After surgery and the resolution of any medical problems, most people want to return home, but many need a period of rehabilitation in order to do so. Few hospitals organise this aspect of care well. Rehabilitation requires careful assessment, planning and evaluation (Exhibit 6) which builds on the care planned and delivered when patients are first admitted.

14. Rehabilitation also requires good teamwork between the many professionals involved. For multidisciplinary working to be effective, someone should have overall responsibility for planning and reviewing the progress of each patient from day to day. While the consultant remains responsible, nurses are well placed to co-ordinate the various professional groups on a day-to-day basis and liaise with the family.

15. There should be clear lines of communication. These might include weekly ward meetings, daily handovers, and joint working with patients to ensure consistency and a patient-centred approach. Good assessment tools assist communication between professionals and provide a basis for evaluation.

16. Rehabilitation may happen in a number of places:

◆ orthopaedic wards

◆ specialist orthogeriatric units

◆ general elderly rehabilitation wards

◆ early supported discharge or hospital-at-home schemes.

17. Simple factors such as clothing, the structure of the day and the ward environment are crucial to a sense of dignity and autonomy. Wherever possible, patients should be encouraged to dress in their own

clothes. A good ward environment provides encouragement, with furniture at the right height, non-slip floors, hand rails, good lighting and signposting, and easy access to personal belongings (Ref. 4).

18. There are real advantages to getting patients home for their rehabilitation, but hospital-at-home schemes must be well organised and have sufficient resources if they are to work effectively and safely.

Exhibit 6
The rehabilitation cycle

Careful assessment, planning and evaluation are required.

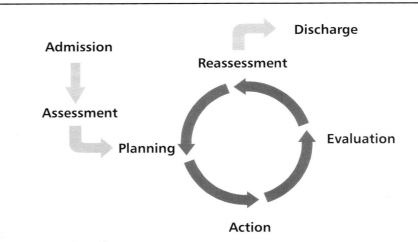

*'If other aspects of care
are planned properly,
good discharge follows
as a natural
consequence'*

and
the return home

19. Discharge home is the final stage of the patient's hospital stay. If the other aspects of care, from admission, through acute care to rehabilitation are planned properly, good discharge follows as a natural consequence. If any part is skimped, the consequences emerge at discharge.

20. Various steps are needed during the course of treatment if discharge is to proceed smoothly:

◆ identification of people likely to need help after discharge;

◆ early specification of a target date for discharge;

◆ full assessment and planning of the support needed at home (which is likely to include a home visit as the target date approaches);

◆ full involvement of patients and their relatives throughout the process;

◆ organisation of the support required; and

◆ monitoring of the progress towards discharge and any causes of delay.

The process needs to bring together professionals from hospital, community health, and social services.

21. As with the admission process, a good way of ensuring that planning takes place is through routine documentation. As part of this study, patient records were examined for evidence of discharge planning. The results were generally poor (Exhibit 7).

Exhibit 7
Discharge planning documentation

Documentation was generally poor.

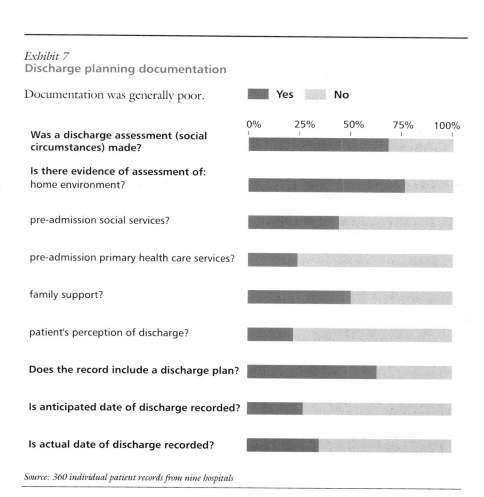

Source: 360 individual patient records from nine hospitals

wider lessons

'Many of the principles could equally be applied to elderly patients with other conditions'

22. Many of the lessons learned from this study could be applied more widely. Purchasers could start to specify some of the good practices described in this report (Exhibit 8). And many of the principles could equally well be applied to elderly patients with other conditions.

23. It is also important to involve patients and their relatives fully throughout the process. Many do not feel sufficiently involved. Full involvement is crucial if patients are to return home safely.

References

1. Royal College of Physicians, *Fractured Neck of Femur: Prevention and Management*, RCP, 1989

2. British Orthopaedics Association, *The Management of Skeletal Trauma in the UK*, BOA, 1992

3. E A Campling, H B Devlin, R W Hoile, J N Lunn, *The Report of the National Confidential Enquiry into Perioperative Deaths 1990*, NCEPOD, 1992

4. The British Geriatrics Society, the Royal College of Psychiatrists and the Royal College of Nursing, *Improving Care of Elderly People in Hospital*, 1987

Exhibit 8
A list of good practice

Purchasers could start to specify some of the good practices described in this report.

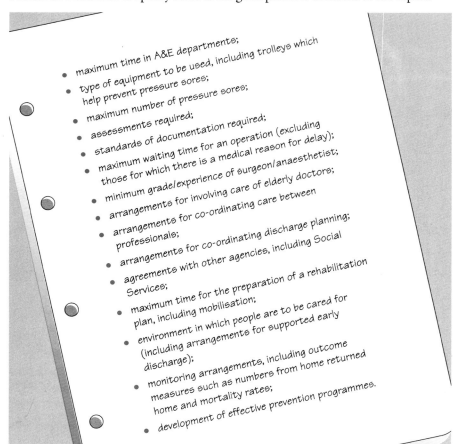

- maximum time in A&E departments;
- type of equipment to be used, including trolleys which help prevent pressure sores;
- maximum number of pressure sores;
- assessments required;
- standards of documentation required;
- maximum waiting time for an operation (excluding those for which there is a medical reason for delay);
- minimum grade/experience of surgeon/anaesthetist;
- arrangements for involving care of elderly doctors;
- arrangements for co-ordinating care between professionals;
- arrangements for co-ordinating discharge planning;
- agreements with other agencies, including Social Services;
- maximum time for the preparation of a rehabilitation plan, including mobilisation;
- environment in which people are to be cared for (including arrangements for supported early discharge);
- monitoring arrangements, including outcome measures such as numbers from home returned home and mortality rates;
- development of effective prevention programmes.

If you want to know more:

The full details of the Audit Commission's study into hip fracture are published in the National Report, *United They Stand: Co-ordinating Care for Elderly Patients with Hip Fracture.*

Published by HMSO
ISBN 011 886434 3
Price £10.00

Telephone orders: 0171-873 9090

The Audit Commission for Local Authorities and the National Health Service in England and Wales, 1 Vincent Square, London SWIP 2PN Tel: 0171 828 1212

Preface

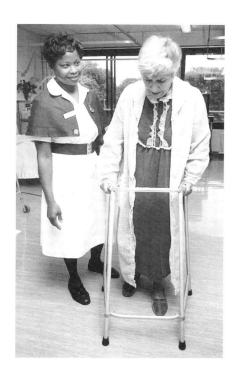

'Our thanks go to all staff who gave so much of their time to the study team.'

The Audit Commission oversees the external audit of local authorities and agencies within the National Health Service (NHS) in England and Wales. As part of its function, the Commission is charged with reviewing the economy, efficiency and effectiveness of services provided by those bodies. To this end, studies and audits of selected topics are undertaken each year.

This study of the care received by elderly people who have fractured a hip examines the process of care up to their discharge from hospital. It focuses on:

◆ the working relationships between different professional groups;

◆ assessment and treatment; and

◆ the arrangements for rehabilitation and return to the community.

The study was carried out at nine hospitals across the country. Our thanks go to all staff who gave so much of their time to the study team. Local audits will take place in all acute hospitals in England and Wales during the next year.

If people are to maintain their independence, what happens after discharge is equally important, particularly the provision of help with mobility and social care, and the continuity of care between hospital and community health services. The Department of Health's Clinical Standards Advisory Group (CSAG) is currently using fractured neck of femur as a tracer condition to study care in the community once patients have been discharged from hospital. The CSAG study teams are visiting the same areas as the Audit Commission. Their recommendations, due to be published in 1996, will build on this report.

This study was carried out by Linda Jarrett, Caroline Gardner and Kay Greenhalgh, under the general direction of Dr Jonathan Boyce and David Browning. Helen Read and Stuart Bailey assisted with data collection and analysis. Eileen Shepherd (nursing consultant), Mr Glyn Prior (consultant orthopaedic surgeon) and Professor Ian Philp (consultant in elderly care medicine) provided additional advice. The study was also supported by an advisory group (Appendix 1). The Audit Commission is grateful to all the individuals and organisations who assisted with this study. Responsibility for the contents and conclusions rests solely with the Audit Commission.

3

Introduction

'The higher estimate [in the growth of the rate of hip fracture] would require extra beds and other resources equivalent to eight new district general hospitals...'

1. Hip fracture poses a significant challenge to health and social services – 57,000 people are affected each year, at an estimated cost of £250 million for hospital care alone. Most people who fracture a hip are elderly; nine out of ten are over 65, and three-quarters are over 75. The majority are women.

2. Most hip fractures result from a fall. The cause of the fall may be unclear, but a number of factors play a part. Illness is a major cause of falls at home, and accidents may be caused by slowed reflexes, dizziness associated with medication or blood pressure problems and environmental hazards. Thinning of the bones with age makes them more likely to break. Extensive research has confirmed how difficult it is to develop effective prevention programmes, although it is now generally accepted that hormone replacement at the time of the menopause may play a part in preventing bones from thinning and hence may help prevent some fractures (Refs. 1, 2).

3. The number of hip fractures is rising, partly because of the growth of the elderly population, but also because the number of people per head of population who fracture a hip (the 'rate' of fracture) is increasing (Ref. 3). In 1989 it was estimated that the growth in population would produce 60,000 cases each year by 2016. The growth in the rate of fracture could increase this number to as many as 117,000 cases. The latest available figures suggest some continuing growth in the rate (Exhibit 1), with the number of new cases over the next 30 years likely to be somewhere between these two estimates.

4. Under current patterns of care, the higher estimate would require extra beds and other resources equivalent to eight new district general hospitals over the next 20 years. Even a more modest growth rate will require considerable extra resources. If the NHS is to be able to cope with this increase within existing resources, it is essential that best practice is adopted as widely as possible, both to maximise the extent to which people recover and minimise

Exhibit 1
Incidence of hip fracture in England and Wales

Latest figures suggest continued growth in the rate of fracture.

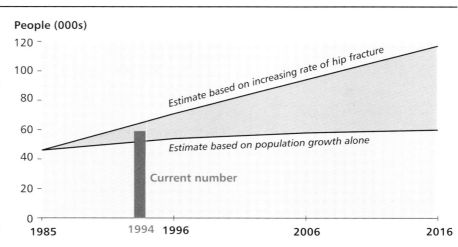

People (000s)

Source: Royal College of Physicians (Ref. 5) Table 4

the resources required for both acute care and continuing care. Considerable progress has been made in recent years in the treatment of patients with a hip fracture, and most fractures can now be repaired surgically. Most patients can walk again within a day or two of surgery, and can be home within a few weeks unless frailty or medical complications cause delays. But effective co-ordination of services is required if care is to be successful, as the process is often complex.

5. Hip fracture patients frequently have other, quite different needs from other orthopaedic patients, and have more in common with patients on elderly care wards. The ageing process inevitably means that many older people become more frail and vulnerable as time passes, and suffer from a number of medical problems that may be complicated by their social circumstances. It is often these illnesses that cause their fall and fracture in the first place. Four in five hip fracture patients suffer from conditions common in old age, such as hypertension, diabetes, dementia or Parkinson's disease. Others develop medical problems while they are in hospital as a consequence of their injury. If these patients are to recover as fully as possible, these other conditions must be treated alongside the hip fracture.

Co-ordinating care

6. Most patients who fracture their hips:

- are admitted to hospital via the nearest accident and emergency department;
- are then transferred to an orthopaedic ward under the care of an orthopaedic surgeon for an operation to repair the fracture;
- receive treatment for medical conditions, often from a physician specialising in the care of the elderly;
- undergo a programme of rehabilitation after their operation, receiving care and treatment from nurses and therapy staff, either on acute wards or in services designed specifically for older patients; and
- return home, or move on to sheltered housing or to permanent residential or nursing home care for the first time (Exhibit 2).

7. During the study, nine hospitals were visited and their patterns of care reviewed. This is a small sample, making it difficult to generalise with any degree of statistical confidence. But the problems identified, and the good practice reported, are likely to be of widespread interest, and they also accord with the findings of other studies (Ref. 4).

8. This report reviews problems found at each stage of the care of elderly hip fracture patients and makes proposals for what can be done to address them. But the over-riding problem is that the separate stages of their treatment are difficult to co-ordinate to provide a cohesive whole: people's needs are rarely considered in the round.

9. Traditionally, the NHS is made up of groups of professionals with separate reporting lines, with full responsibility for people currently in their care and the tasks they are trained to undertake; but most refer on to others once their individual responsibilities have been discharged. This approach can work very

Exhibit 2
The process of care for hip fracture patients

Hip fracture patients use a wide variety of services.

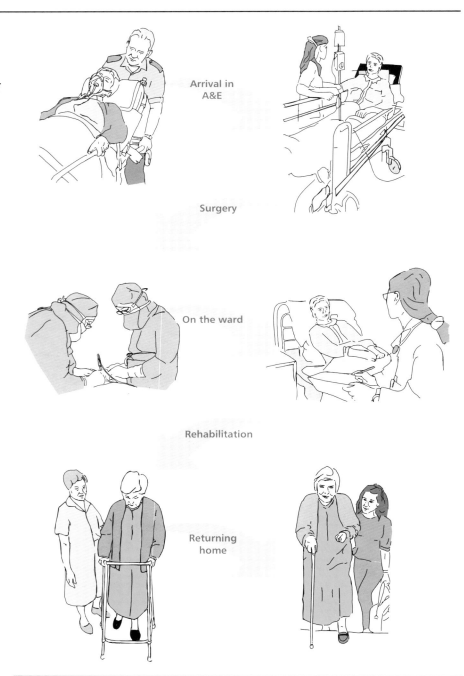

Arrival in A&E

Surgery

On the ward

Rehabilitation

Returning home

Source: Audit Commission

well for patients with straightforward problems that require the involvement of only one or two practitioners; but it is difficult to co-ordinate care for people with multiple problems who frequently require support from different professionals, often from separate agencies. This type of situation, common in community care (and a major cause of difficulty with that policy), also occurs in hospital.

Exhibit 3
Discharge destinations of patients admitted from home

There is a wide variation in the percentage of patients who return directly home.

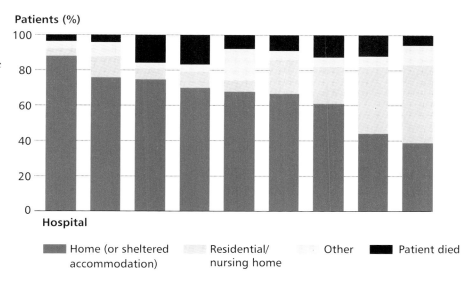

Source: 450 patient records from nine hospitals

10. Most patients do go home after a hip fracture, but the proportion varies significantly between the hospitals studied (Exhibit 3).

11. Some of this variation is no doubt explained by sample size and case mix, as the likelyhood of a return home depends on the frailty and age of the person involved, and on the type and complexity of the fracture. But the size of variation is such that it indicates that hospitals are adopting different approaches. Other studies have shown similar variations between hospitals without significant differences between patients, suggesting that some hospitals are more effective than others. A recent audit of care in hospitals in East Anglia found that people admitted to one of the eight hospitals in the sample had a much lower mortality rate than the others (Exhibit 4, overleaf) (Ref. 4). It would appear that it is the total package of care which affects outcomes rather than any one single factor.

12. The cost of care varies with the intensity of support and length of stay. The average cost of hospital care per case is about £5,000, but this figure conceals a wide variation which is not related to quality. A low cost may result from a speedy recovery following effective treatment, or from a discharge home without sufficient rehabilitation and support. A high cost may result from a careful, thorough rehabilitation programme, or a protracted stay due to a lack of rehabilitation and discharge planning. Hence cost on its own is not a good guide to performance.

13. The Royal College of Physicians has produced recommendations on the effective management of patients who have fractured their hips (Ref. 5 and Appendix 2), and the Royal College of Nursing in conjunction with the British Geriatrics Society and the Royal College of Psychiatrists has produced guidance on improving care of elderly people in hospital (Ref.6). The Audit

Exhibit 4
Different mortality rates from different hospitals

People admitted to one of eight hospitals had a much lower mortality rate than those admitted to the others.

Percentage of patients surviving 90 days following surgery for fractured hip

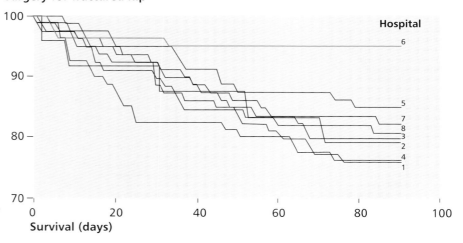

Source: British Medical Journal, Vol. 310 (6984), p907 (C J Todd, C J Freeman, C Camilleri-Ferrant et al, 'Differences in mortality after fracture of hip: The East Anglian audit')

Commission has used these guidelines to assess the care of patients at the nine hospitals visited, and to identify the arrangements which help to meet the standards set.

Patients' views

14. As part of this study, a group of hip fracture patients were interviewed about their experiences by the College of Health, an organisation experienced in patient opinion research. Patients, their relatives and other carers talked to researchers about the care they received while in hospital and on discharge. This confirmed the findings of previous Audit Commission research – patients and carers do not always receive the information they need, and they may receive conflicting information from the different professionals involved in their care. Patients' comments are used throughout the report to illustrate particular aspects of care.

Overview

The report is divided into four chapters. The first three follow the progress of patients through the hospital as outlined in Exhibit 2, and the fourth draws some wider lessons.

1 **Chapter 1** examines what happens when patients are first admitted to hospital. Delays are common in accident and emergency departments (A&E), requiring a streamlining of procedures. Assessment of people's circumstances should start in A&E and continue after admission to the orthopaedic ward, to provide the basis for planning subsequent treatment and care.

2 **Chapter 2** describes the treatment patients receive. Nearly all hip fractures are treated surgically; hospitals need to check that people do not wait longer than necessary for surgery and that operations are performed by doctors with sufficient experience. Many elderly people would also benefit from the attention of an elderly care doctor because they suffer from other medical conditions. Hospitals vary in the extent to which such doctors are involved. While no single model of liaison stands out, it is important that responsibility for taking the lead and co-ordinating care is clear and unambiguous.

3 **Chapter 3** examines the process of rehabilitation and the return home. Most patients need a period of rehabilitation after surgery, which requires good teamwork between the many professionals involved. While people who were fit before fracturing their hips can expect effective rehabilitation schemes in most hospitals, co-ordination is frequently poor for those who are more frail and whose recovery is likely to take longer. Early discharge schemes that get patients home with extensive support appear to be particularly effective if well managed – but discharge requires early identification of those requiring help and good co-ordination to plan the help needed. Few hospitals, however, start discharge planning early enough, resulting in long waits and other problems.

4 **Chapter 4** draws out the wider lessons for the hospital care of elderly people in general. Many of the lessons from this study of hip fracture, described above, apply equally to the care of elderly people with other conditions. Most experience admission through A&E, full assessment, treatment requiring care from different doctors, and rehabilitation and discharge home with care from different professionals and agencies. And all elderly people and their carers need to be informed and consulted at every stage of their care and treatment.

5   **The need for co-ordinated care** is common to many elderly people (and indeed to others in younger age groups) with complex conditions requiring the involvement of different groups of professionals from different agencies over an extended period of time. In each case, someone must take overall responsibility, supported by appropriate tools to help co-ordination proceed smoothly. Purchasers should provide a lead, setting out requirements within contracts; and hospitals need to allocate responsibilities and establish a system for recording information in ways which provide a link between professionals. The 'care programme approach' developed for those with mental health problems offers one model.

6   **Solutions to these challenges** are becoming ever more urgent as the number of elderly people in the population grows, with a 60 per cent increase in those over 65 and a doubling of those over 85 projected in the next 30 years. Pressures on health and social services are likely to grow significantly as a result. This report and the programme of local audits planned for England and Wales are intended to help authorities and trusts start planning ways of ensuring that elderly people receive the care and support they need, both now and in the future.

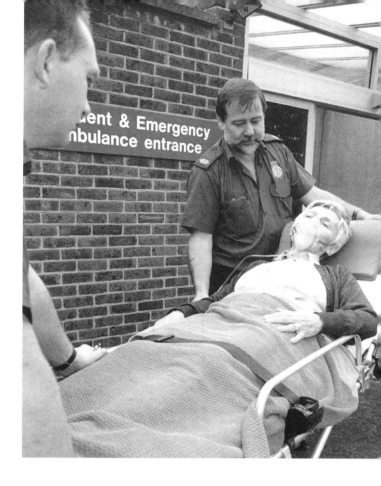

1 Admission

Almost all patients with fractured hips are admitted through accident and emergency (A&E) departments. Too many spend too long in these departments. Better procedures are needed to speed up their admission to wards.

More extensive assessment of people's circumstances is also needed, to identify current difficulties more systematically and to provide a basis for planning treatment and care.

15. When an elderly person with a fractured hip arrives at hospital, the immediate priorities are:

◆ to confirm the diagnosis and assess his or her medical, nursing and social needs so that care can be planned effectively; and

◆ to fix the fracture securely so that rehabilitation can begin as soon as possible.

This chapter considers the actions which need to take place, first in the A&E department and then in orthopaedic trauma wards, to tackle the first of these priorities.

Accident and emergency

16. Almost all patients who have fractured their hips are admitted via A&E departments. The only exceptions are patients who fracture a hip while already in hospital for some other reason, and patients admitted to the few hospitals which have a specific arrangement in place to bypass A&E (perhaps because the orthopaedic trauma wards are on a separate site).

17. A number of routine procedures take place when someone with a suspected hip fracture arrives, and in most hospitals they occur, or at least begin, in A&E (Exhibit 5). Some procedures are concerned with diagnosing the fracture; others are necessary to start addressing the wider needs of older patients. The challenge to staff is to achieve both efficiently and effectively.

18. The Patient's Charter states that all patients should receive an initial assessment within five minutes of arrival in A&E. Many departments meet this standard, but patients often then wait several hours for a full assessment and treatment, especially if their problem is not perceived to be urgent. The Royal College of Physicians' guidelines recommend that hip fracture patients should not spend more than one hour in A&E.

19. This recommendation is important because many elderly hip fracture patients arriving in A&E have often already spent some time undiscovered on the floor at home. Because of the changes associated with ageing, this leaves them vulnerable to pain, confusion and dehydration, all of which may result in longer stays and poorer outcomes.

20. In addition, older patients are particularly vulnerable to pressure sores, which can start to develop in as little as 30 minutes and may already be present when the patient is admitted. It can be difficult to offer proper pressure area care in A&E due to staff workloads and a lack of equipment. Only one hospital had equipment that allowed patients to be x-rayed on a soft surface. However pressure sore risk should always be assessed as soon as possible in A&E and immediate prevention and care carried out.

Exhibit 5
The routine in A&E

A number of routine procedures take place when someone with a suspected hip fracture arrives:

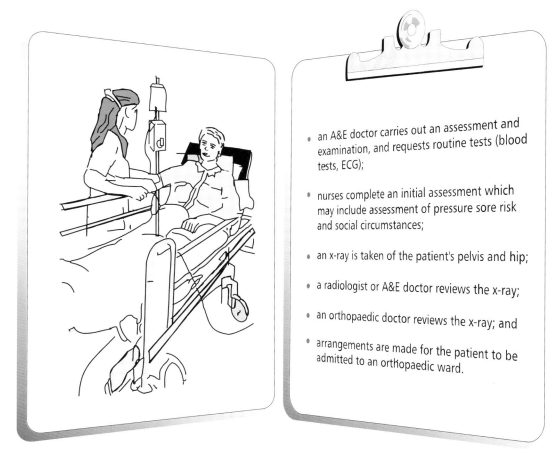

- an A&E doctor carries out an assessment and examination, and requests routine tests (blood tests, ECG);

- nurses complete an initial assessment which may include assessment of pressure sore risk and social circumstances;

- an x-ray is taken of the patient's pelvis and hip;

- a radiologist or A&E doctor reviews the x-ray;

- an orthopaedic doctor reviews the x-ray; and

- arrangements are made for the patient to be admitted to an orthopaedic ward.

Source: Audit Commission

21. Staff in all of the hospitals visited agreed in principle with the RCP recommendation, but most patients waited longer than an hour (Exhibit 6, overleaf).

22. Most A&E departments do not have accurate records of the factors which contribute to long waits. There are several points at which delays may occur: people may have to wait before seeing a doctor, before having an x-ray, and then again while their x-ray is being assessed. And staff in A&E departments commented on the wait for an orthopaedic doctor to arrive to confirm the fracture and arrange the patient's admission to the ward.

Exhibit 6
Length of time patients spend in A&E

Most patients wait longer than one hour.

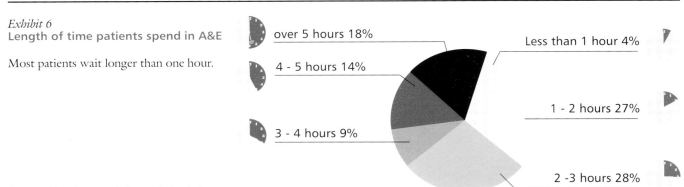

over 5 hours 18%

4 - 5 hours 14%

3 - 4 hours 9%

Less than 1 hour 4%

1 - 2 hours 27%

2 -3 hours 28%

Source: 400 patient records from eight hospitals

23. In many cases, orthopaedic doctors work in operating theatres or clinics while on call, and patients in A&E have to wait until they are free. But some hospitals make special arrangements to avoid this problem (Case Study 1), either by ensuring that the orthopaedic doctor on call is available or by introducing procedures to be followed if no one is available.

"The biggest hassle was lying there, nobody tells you anything, they're all dashing about."

24. Many patients find busy A&E departments overwhelming and older people are particularly vulnerable. Hospitals vary in the provisions they make for dealing with elderly people, including those with a hip fracture (Exhibit 7). Most A&E departments do not have immediate access to expertise in elderly care or social care assessment. While no particular combination of services has been shown to make a decisive difference and it may be unrealistic to expect all of them to be provided, hospitals should nevertheless review their arrangements for caring for elderly people in A&E departments to see how they can be improved.

Case Study 1
Arrangements to speed older patients through A&E

At Peterborough District Hospital the junior orthopaedic doctors do not work in theatres when on call. This means that they are free to attend A&E when necessary; as a result, patients wait less time before they are transferred to the ward.

Hastings and Rother NHS Trust has written guidelines for the early management of hip fracture patients, designed to reduce waits and the risk of pressure sores.

◆ Patients with fractured neck of femur are placed in a high priority group;

◆ Pressure-relieving equipment is placed under pressure areas;

◆ Following examination, but prior to x-ray, analgesia is administered when required. The use of femoral nerve blocks is encouraged;

◆ Patients are reviewed promptly on return from x-ray;

◆ If the diagnosis is confirmed the orthopaedic SHO/house officer is notified and arrangements are made to transfer the patient to the ward without delay;

◆ If the orthopaedic doctor anticipates a delay in attending to the patient on the ward, the Accident Officer initiates intravenous fluids prior to the patient's transfer from the A&E department; and

◆ Patients are clerked in on the ward and not in the A&E department. Patients are only reviewed in A&E if there is some doubt about the diagnosis.

Exhibit 7
A&E services for older patients

Hospitals vary in the provision they make for dealing with elderly people.

Provision in nine hospitals

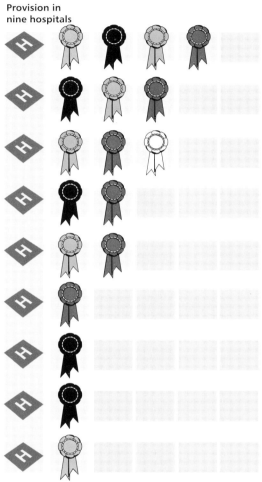

A nurse specifically trained in the care of older people

A social worker available full time

Arrangements for following up progress of patients discharged from A&E

Notification of the patient's GP by A&E staff

Periodic audit of the causes of falls

Provision for elderly people

Source: Audit Commission

"I didn't have to wait five minutes, they took me into a little room straight away, and I had four or five nurses, and they never left me ...and they were asking me questions about everything and ... doing blood tests: they were wonderful.."

25. Without early assessment vital information may be missed. People arriving at A&E are often accompanied by a friend, relative or neighbour who can provide extra information; and ambulance staff are often able to comment on home circumstances. Wherever possible, this information should be recorded and either acted upon immediately, or passed on to others who will be responsible for planning the eventual programme of rehabilitation. For example, immediate action is needed where patients are caring for someone older and frailer than themselves at home. Hospital staff must ensure that the necessary community services are alerted to take over from the carer while she or he is in hospital.

On to the ward

26. Because of their complex needs, hip fracture patients need a full assessment of their medical, nursing and social problems. This assessment, started within the A&E department, needs to be completed once they reach the ward (with some of the main components set out in Box A, overleaf).

27. The initial assessment in A&E normally involves nurses assessing pressure sore risk and asking a few key questions about the patient's social circumstances, as discussed in the previous section.

Assessment

28. Even though many of their patients are elderly, staff on orthopaedic wards have not necessarily been trained in the care of elderly people; the emphasis is on safely preparing patients for surgery. This means that assessment is sometimes incomplete. If hip fracture patients are not fully assessed, problems may arise which directly affect their well-being, either immediately in preparation for surgery or in the longer term, during recovery. The consequences of incomplete assessment may include:

◆ **Delays in operation**

– Medical conditions may go undiagnosed until just before the operation, which then has to be cancelled; and

– Deficiencies in hydration or nutrition may themselves contribute to delayed operations and may also lead to other serious conditions.

◆ **Misdiagnosis**

– Older patients may be temporarily confused, either before the operation as a result of pain or the injury itself, or afterwards as a result of the anaesthetic or medication. This confusion may be incorrectly diagnosed as dementia, leading to inappropriate treatment in the short term, and inappropriate planning for the longer term; and

– Incontinence may be mismanaged because nurses have inadequate knowledge of the causes of incontinence and its treatment. The use of an in-dwelling catheter in preference to more labour-intensive, though often better, methods of promoting continence may lead to other problems, such as discomfort, loss of independence and dignity, and possibly infection.

◆ **Delays in recovery and discharge**

– Failure to assess and treat pain means that patients suffer unnecessarily and may take longer to recover;

– If patients develop pressure sores, their lengths of stay are likely to increase significantly and their chance of full recovery may be reduced;

– Post-operative plans for rehabilitation may be unrealistic if nurses and therapists lack full information about patients' previous functional ability; and

– If patients' social circumstances are not fully assessed on admission, delays may occur in addressing problems once they are fit and ready to go home.

'Because of their complex needs, hip fracture patients need a full assessment of their medical, nursing and social problems.'

29. Each ward should have standard nursing documentation which includes prompts for the main components of assessment on admission, and assessment tools giving an objective measure of problems as recommended by the Royal College of Nursing (Ref. 7), the Royal College of Physicians and the British Geriatrics Society (Ref. 8). Some hospitals do not have such documentation and, even where they do, nurses do not always complete the forms (Exhibit 8).

30. At the hospitals visited there was often a lack of detail about patients' individual needs and problems in the nursing notes. For example, most assessments of nutrition failed to consider risk factors such as ill-fitting false teeth, mouth infections, or inability to handle cutlery, and concentrated instead on information about foods disliked by patients. Many using the forms seemed to have difficulty in deciding what information to record and where.

Exhibit 8
Standard nursing documentation of assessment on admission

Even when forms include prompts for assessment, they are sometimes not completed.

Yes
No

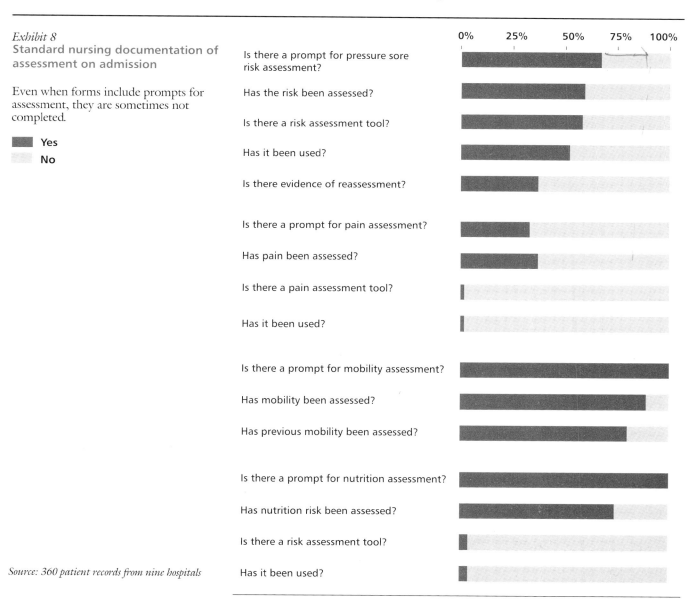

Is there a prompt for pressure sore risk assessment?

Has the risk been assessed?

Is there a risk assessment tool?

Has it been used?

Is there evidence of reassessment?

Is there a prompt for pain assessment?

Has pain been assessed?

Is there a pain assessment tool?

Has it been used?

Is there a prompt for mobility assessment?

Has mobility been assessed?

Has previous mobility been assessed?

Is there a prompt for nutrition assessment?

Has nutrition risk been assessed?

Is there a risk assessment tool?

Has it been used?

Source: 360 patient records from nine hospitals

Box A
Some of the main
components of an
assessment for older
patients

Pressure sore risk

Age-related changes in the skin increase the risk of skin breakdown. A frail older person may experience damage in as little as 30 minutes. A validated risk assessment tool highlights the risk factors for pressure sores:

- female, aged 75 or over;
- dehydration;
- underweight;
- debilitating disorders;
- poor nutrition;
- trauma and surgery;
- reduced mobility;
- pain;
- discoloured or broken skin; and
- poorly managed continence.

The specific risk factors can then be addressed through a plan of care.

Hydration and nutrition

In addition to a straightforward assessment of hydration, the patient's nutritional risk factors should be considered. Nutritional status can be affected by physical, social and economic constraints:

- impaired taste and smell can lead to loss of appetite;
- ill-fitting dentures or oral infections can cause soreness of the mouth and gums ;
- Parkinson's tremor, poor sight and poor co-ordination make it difficult for people to feed themselves in unfamiliar surroundings;
- poverty limits the food that people can afford;
- depression, bereavement, social isolation and loneliness may take away the motivation to prepare food and eat; and
- confusion and dementia may cause the patient to forget to eat.

Pain

In the past, assessment of pain has often been based on the subjective judgement of nurse and patient (and many older patients do not like to 'make a fuss'), but a variety of pain assessment tools now exist which aim to provide a more objective measure of pain. The benefits include:

- more accurate information on the level of pain;
- information to help establish the pattern of pain;
- evaluation of the effects of medication; and
- a framework for setting specific goals.

For some elderly patients the pain of the fracture may add to chronic pain associated with other conditions. Each problem should be assessed carefully, as different care may be required.

Continence

Incontinence is a symptom of an underlying problem, and a thorough assessment is needed. The causes of incontinence can include constipation, urinary infection, pelvic floor damage or neurological disease, and each requires a different plan of care.

Co-existing medical problems

The patient's past medical history may include illness that could affect anaesthesia, including respiratory and cardiac disorders. A drug history is also useful. Patients and carers should both be involved in this assessment; useful information can also be obtained from the GP or district nurse and, perhaps, social services. The assessment should also cover the patient's overall well-being. Vague symptoms may indicate problems with long-term use of sedatives or other drugs, or undiagnosed medical problems.

Mental state

Poor cognitive function is closely associated with poor outcome following a hospital stay. Confusion due to pain, dehydration or simple disorientation can be misdiagnosed as dementia, so a careful assessment is necessary to ensure that the right care is provided. Simple tools are available which give a guide to cognitive function, such as the geriatric depression score and the mini mental state examination. The person's lifestyle and past history are important; someone who has recently developed acute confusion requires very different care from an elderly person with long-term memory loss. Early (and full) involvement of the person's carer is important.

Previous mobility

In older people, mobility is often more important than diagnosis in predicting outcomes. Assessment of previous mobility provides a baseline against which realistic goals can be set and progress measured:

- how far could the patient walk?
- could the patient climb stairs?
- what aids were required?
- did they become breathless?

Again, consultation with somebody who knows the person well may produce more realistic and reliable results.

Functional ability

This includes an assessment of how an individual carries out the activities that fitter people take for granted. The assessment should include:

- the patient's normal routine;
- what they do for recreation;
- how they wash and dress;
- their interests and hobbies; and
- how they prepare food;
- any paid employment.

Things the patient is no longer able to do should be considered, such as visiting friends, bathing or cooking. This allows the development of a plan to address problems.

Social circumstances

The assessment should include:

- the condition of the patient's home and their ability to function in that environment;
- their financial circumstances, including any problems with pensions or bills; and
- support from family, friends, and others such as district nurses or home-helps. The discussion should include the individual's preferences for the future, the views of carers and relatives, and what they think they can cope with realistically.

Source: Audit Commission

When prompts for the assessment of problems such as pain were absent, nothing was recorded on the assessment form or the care plan.

31. Where assessment and care planning is of poor quality, many important factors are not taken into consideration. It is also harder for staff to develop individual care plans, and for staff taking over responsibility to know what has happened before.

32. Information should not only be obtained from the patient. Patients should in turn be provided with good information at all stages about what is happening to them, why, and what is likely to happen in the future. Many are shocked and frightened and need reassurance. One hospital had produced a clearly printed card which gave clear information to everyone with a hip fracture.

33. Wherever possible, information should be given to the patient and carer or relative together. Messages can get distorted in their retelling, raising anxieties and causing unnecessary difficulties which may impede successful rehabilitation after the operation.

Pressure area care

34. The high incidence of pressure sores reinforces the importance of systematic assessment. Pressure sores are a particular problem for elderly patients with fractured hips, because of their age, their immobility, and the frailty of many. They cause pain and discomfort, require special equipment and intensive nursing care, and lead to longer hospital stays, costing an estimated £320 million in 1993. But most pressure sores are preventable and, for a high-risk group like elderly hip fracture patients, prevention is both cost-effective and improves the quality of care immeasurably.

35. The Department of Health has highlighted the incidence of pressure sores as a key quality indicator, and purchasers and providers are required to set annual targets for reducing their prevalence. The incidence of pressure sores in elective orthopaedic wards has been estimated to be 2.7 per cent, but in trauma wards it can be as high as 42.7 per cent (Ref. 9).

36. Some hip fracture patients develop sores while lying on the floor at home after their fall, but others develop them in hospital because they do not receive adequate preventative care. There is sometimes a lack of understanding about the aim of pressure sore risk assessment. At hospitals visited during the study, nurses often said that they assess patients they consider to be at risk, missing the point that the aim of the assessment is to identify systematically those patients who are at risk, and to indicate the preventative action required. To prevent pressure sores, nurses must use risk assessment tools consistently and act on the results.

'Pressure sores are a particular problem for elderly patients with fractured hips, because of their age, their immobility, and the frailty of many.'

37. Few hospitals have adopted a comprehensive approach to pressure area care (Exhibit 9). Research has shown that the incidence and prevalence of pressure sores can be reduced with little or no additional expenditure by concentrating on education and training, and by collecting information about the incidence of pressure sores and feeding it back to all staff (Ref. 10). Major improvements have been realised at the Queen's Medical Centre, Nottingham for example (Case Study 2, overleaf).

Exhibit 9
Approaches to pressure sore prevention

Few hospitals have adopted a comprehensive approach to pressure area care.

Provision in nine hospitals

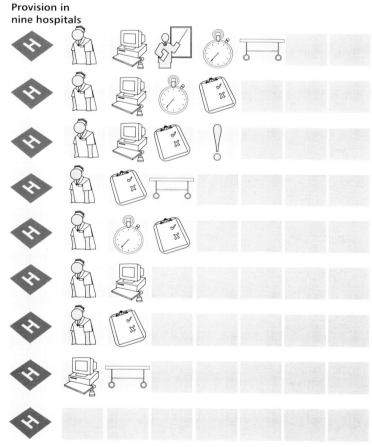

Characteristics of pressure area care

 Clear responsibility

 Incidence/prevalence data collected

 Staff informed of results

 Standard times for assessment

 Hospital-wide assessment system

 Equipment audit

 A&E staff assume all hip fracture patients are at risk

Source: Audit Commission

'Wherever possible, information should be given to the patient and carer or relative together.'

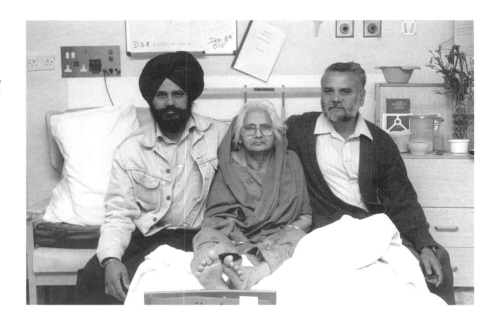

Case Study 2
Sigma project, Queen's Medical Centre

The aims of this project were:

◆ to collect data about the incidence of pressure sores; and

◆ to reduce the incidence of hospital-acquired sores to zero.

The project applied to all patients aged 70 years and over admitted to two pilot Health Care of the Elderly wards, via A&E and the hospital's GP Unit .

The following process was adopted:

◆ Patients admitted through A&E have a risk assessment carried out within five minutes of arriving in the department;

◆ Patients with planned admission to the ward have a risk assessment carried out within 30 minutes of admission;

◆ Pressure-relieving equipment is provided for those patients assessed as being at risk of developing pressure sores. Equipment specific to their needs is provided within two hours;

◆ Pressure-relieving equipment is maintained in a state of readiness;

◆ Patients assessed as being at risk have their needs evaluated within their care programmes; and

◆ Patients and their carers receive a formal programme of education and advice regarding pressure sore prevention and treatment.

The incidence of hospital-acquired pressure sores for the pilot wards fell from 19 per cent before the project started to 2 per cent six months later. An economic evaluation showed that this reduction was achieved at nominal cost.

Recommendations

Managers and doctors in acute hospitals should work together to:

1 audit the time spent by hip fracture patients in A&E, and identify the reasons for delays in transferring patients to the wards;

2 bring A&E, radiology and orthopaedic staff together to review ways of speeding patients through the department, and agree:
- a waiting time standard for elderly patients in A&E, and
- procedures for the management of hip fracture patients on admission;

3 review arrangements for caring for elderly people within A&E departments;

4 ensure that all patients are assessed within an agreed time for pressure sore risk, and receive the necessary preventive care; and

5 monitor these standards to see that they are met in practice.

They should enhance the standard of assessment for elderly patients by:

6 reviewing the content of standard nursing documentation on orthopaedic wards and other wards admitting elderly patients;

7 revising the documentation if necessary, to ensure that it includes prompts for assessment in each key area, using risk assessment tools;

8 providing ongoing training to nursing staff on the use of the documentation and the implications for care; and by

9 auditing the use of the documentation in practice.

They should aim to reduce the incidence of pressure sores by:

10 reviewing pressure area care policies and procedures;

11 developing systems to provide routine information on incidence and prevalence;

12 auditing the use of assessment tools;

13 identifying and meeting training needs; and by

14 ensuring that sufficient pressure relieving equipment is available.

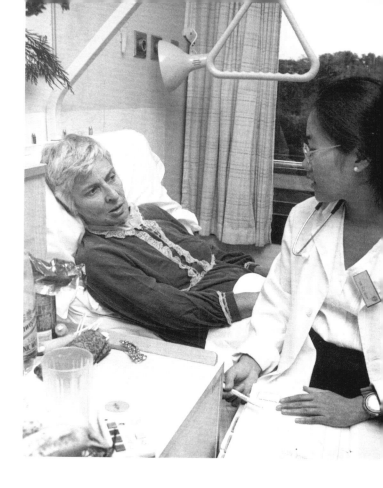

2 Treatment

Treatment involves both surgical and medical care. Nearly all hip fractures are repaired surgically. In some hospitals, operations are performed by unsupervised junior doctors. All hospitals should check that such operations are being carried out by staff with sufficient skills and experience. Some people wait too long for their operations, increasing their discomfort and risk, and tying up resources unnecessarily.

Many older people suffer from other conditions which need medical attention, and some have complex social problems. Physicians specialising in the care of elderly people can help, but hospitals vary in the extent to which they involve them and make use of their skills in the care of hip fracture patients. While no single model for organising medical care stands out, it is important that arrangements are clear and unambiguous, with someone taking overall responsibility for all aspects of care.

Surgical care

38. More than 95 per cent of hip fracture patients have an operation to repair the fracture. Surgery usually involves fixing the fracture with screws and plates, or replacing part of the hip with a metal prosthesis (hemiarthroplasty). Although these are common operations, they require technical skill and experience if they are to be successful, especially where the bone is in poor condition. Operating on elderly patients also requires extra skill, especially in anaesthesia, to take account of pre-existing medical conditions.

39. The aim of the operation is to fix the fracture securely so that rehabilitation can begin as soon as possible. This is more likely to occur if the operation is carried out by experienced doctors (Ref. 11). The Royal College of Physicians' guidelines recommend that these operations should be carried out by experienced doctors.

40. This study found variation in the grade of surgeons and anaesthetists performing hip fracture repairs. Very few had consultant-led operating lists and, although experienced senior doctors usually took responsibility, operations were in some cases carried out by senior house officers (SHOs) without supervision. One operation in ten was carried out by an unsupervised SHO surgeon working with an unsupervised SHO anaesthetist (Exhibit 10). While some SHOs may have sufficient experience to carry out these operations successfully, medical audit should check that the variation observed is properly explained.

Delayed operations

41. If they are medically fit to undergo surgery, hip fracture patients should have their operations as soon as possible. Otherwise:

◆ patients may become distressed and anxious about the delay;

◆ they may take longer to regain their mobility after the operation;

◆ complications such as pressure sores or chest infection may occur, further delaying the operation;

◆ patients may experience a lot of pain which may go unassessed and untreated; and

◆ they may find it difficult to eat and to pass urine while lying in bed, leading to further complications.

'Operating on elderly patients requires extra skill, especially in anaesthesia, to take account of pre-existing medical conditions.'

Exhibit 10
Grades of doctors carrying out hip fracture operations

Many operations are carried out by junior surgeons without supervision...

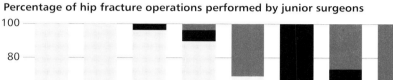
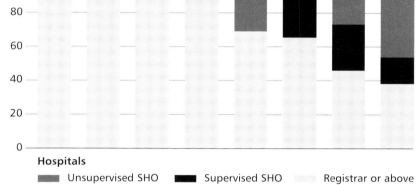

Percentage of hip fracture operations performed by junior surgeons

Hospitals

Unsupervised SHO   Supervised SHO   Registrar or above

...or by unsupervised junior anaesthetists ...

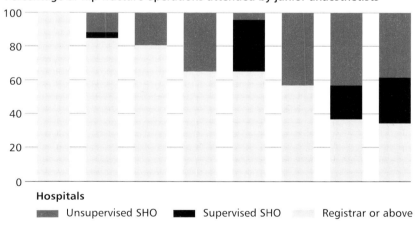

Percentage of hip fracture operations attended by junior anaesthetists

Hospitals

Unsupervised SHO   Supervised SHO   Registrar or above

...and 10 per cent of operations were carried out by two unsupervised juniors working together.

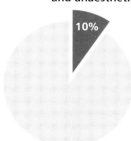

Unsupervised SHO surgeon and anaesthetist

10%

*Source: Records of 220 operations at eight hospitals.
Data unavailable for the ninth hospital visited.*

Exhibit 11
Waits for surgery

Many patients wait longer than one day.

Percentage of patients waiting

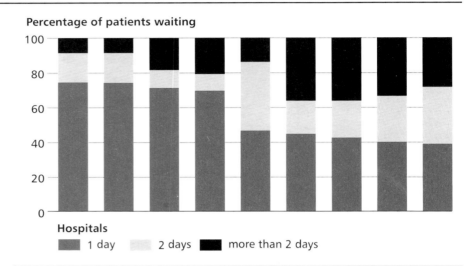

Hospitals

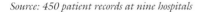

■ 1 day   ▨ 2 days   ■ more than 2 days

Source: 450 patient records at nine hospitals

42. A direct link exists between delayed operations and increased mortality and morbidity (Refs. 4, 12). The Royal College of Physicians recommends that operations should be carried out within 24 hours.

43. In recent years most orthopaedic departments, in negotiation with other theatre users and theatre managers, have attempted to overcome long waits for surgery for hip fracture patients. But there is still a great deal of variation in how long patients wait (Exhibit 11).

44. The ability to operate within 24 hours depends largely on the availability of daily trauma lists. In spite of a long-standing recommendation from the British Orthopaedic Association (Ref. 13), not all hospitals have them. All the hospitals studied for this report schedule some daytime trauma lists, but only two provided them at weekends, probably because there are no elective lists at weekends. This means that a patient admitted with a fractured hip on Friday may not go to theatre until Monday. Some operations are still performed as emergencies at night (Ref. 14), so increasing mortality rates (Ref. 15).

45. A thorough review of theatre use and staffing by managers is the first step in establishing daily trauma lists. At the Conquest Hospital in Hastings, the theatre manager was able to divert resources from emergency night sessions to a scheduled day-time emergency theatre list, with time allocated to orthopaedics.

46. But speed is not everything. In certain circumstances it may be better for a patient to wait more than 24 hours for an operation if it means that an experienced surgeon is then available. When such a delay is planned, precautions can be taken to prevent deterioration in the patient's medical condition. This means information to make sure that the patient knows what is happening, and attention to diet, physiotherapy, pain control and intravenous fluids.

"The nurse said something ... about we can operate on the same night, and then they said we'd have to put it off until tomorrow, and then it was cancelled until Friday ... then they said they weren't certain, they cancelled it on the Friday morning."

"I thought it was a bit much: I'd gone two days on two cups of tea."

47. The problems caused by delay may be compounded unnecessarily by outdated practice in denying patients food and water before surgery. The length of time for which food and drink are withheld is important. Research has shown that a four-hour period is usually sufficient. But in some hospitals food is withheld by routine; patients scheduled for surgery in the morning are starved from midnight, those scheduled for the afternoon list from 6 am. Patients on a morning list may be starved for up to 12 hours.

48. To minimise the risk of dehydration, water and food should be denied for no more than four to six hours, calculated individually for each patient by counting back from the time of operation. The nurse should help to reduce the patient's level of anxiety and confusion by ensuring they understand why they may not eat or drink. If food and drink are withheld for more than eight hours, intravenous fluids should be given. Good liaison between the surgeon, theatre staff and ward staff will ensure that delays are anticipated so that the necessary remedial action can be taken.

49. Despite the importance of early surgery for hip fracture patients, some operations are cancelled at short notice. For elderly patients in particular, repeated starvation can lead to dehydration and nutrition problems, increasing the likelihood of complications and poor recovery. On the orthopaedic wards studied, some patients experienced repeated cancellations at short notice; in some cases nurses reported that this happened at least once a week.

50. In the nine hospitals studied, the total number of 'extra' days in excess of the initial 24 hours for which hip fracture patients awaited surgery amounted to 4,000 each year; the number of days lost was not necessarily linked to the total number of patients (Exhibit 12). While this represents only one or two days per patient, these beds were effectively wasted, since they offered no benefit to the hip fracture patients themselves, and were unavailable to other patients. Eliminating unnecessary waits for surgery would go some way towards releasing the resources needed to meet the demand for extra beds for projected increases in the numbers of people with fractured hips.

Exhibit 12
Bed days lost in waiting for surgery

The number of days lost is not necessarily linked to the total number of patients.

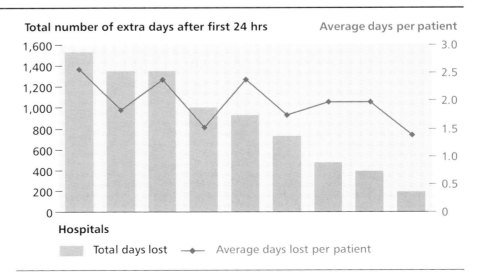

Total number of extra days after first 24 hrs   Average days per patient

Hospitals

Total days lost ◆ Average days lost per patient

Source: 450 patient records at nine hospitals

Medical care

51. Many older people suffer from conditions for which they need medical care, in addition to an operation for their fracture. Indeed, these conditions may have caused the fall and fracture in the first place. Some people also have complex social problems, which must also be addressed if they are to return home successfully. As a result, many could benefit from the specialist skills of elderly care physicians and their teams. In some hospitals there is a close working relationship between orthopaedic surgeons and elderly care physicians, commonly referred to as 'orthogeriatric liaison'. This may take a number of forms, varying from no formal arrangements to close involvement from admission onwards (Box B).

Box B
Models of orthogeriatric liaison

No formal arrangements

Orthopaedic teams take responsibility for all surgical and medical care; the senior house officer commonly takes day to day responsibility. If specialist medical advice is needed, it may be obtained from the general physician on call, rather than an elderly care specialist. A referral to an elderly care consultant for rehabilitation or long-term care tends to be made only if a patient is 'blocking' an orthopaedic bed. This may lead to delays in getting a patient transferred to elderly care or rehabilitation beds.

A named, elderly care doctor liaises with orthopaedics

The elderly care doctor may see all older patients after recovery from the operation, or take selected referrals made by the orthopaedic surgeons. There is usually routine contact, with the elderly care doctor visiting the orthopaedic ward once or twice a week.

The care of older patients may remain the responsibility of the orthopaedic surgeon, with the elderly care physician continuing to give advice and share treatment. In due course patients may be transferred to an elderly care ward when the orthopaedic problem is resolved, or if rehabilitation is expected to take a long time.

Alternatively, responsibility may be transferred to the elderly care physician after initial recovery from surgery. The orthopaedic surgeon may maintain an interest and visit patients until they are discharged, or, more usually, may transfer patients to an elderly care ward or a special rehabilitation ward and not see them again unless an orthopaedic problem develops.

Elderly care physicians are involved in the care of all elderly orthopaedic patients from the time they are admitted

The elderly care doctor may be involved from the start, reviewing medical problems and social circumstances before the operation takes place. Both can then be addressed very early in the discharge planning process, and are explicitly acknowledged as important areas needing the specialist skills of elderly care physicians. Formal arrangements ensure that they are involved routinely.

Exhibit 13
Orthogeriatric liaison at study sites

In some hospitals, surgeons and elderly care physicians work closely.

Hospitals

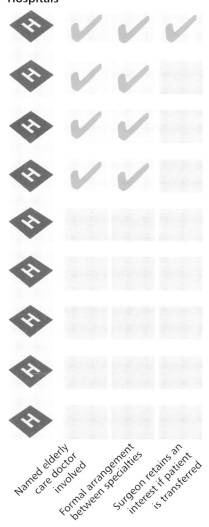

Named elderly care doctor involved

Formal arrangement between specialties

Surgeon retains an interest if patient is transferred

Source: Audit Commission

52. The arrangements for orthogeriatric liaisons at the hospitals studied varied greatly (Exhibit 13).

53. There is some evidence that patients recover more quickly, and are more likely to go back to their previous homes, when the orthogeriatric links are strong (Ref. 16). This is borne out by data from study sites, which suggest that where there is some formal liaison between orthopaedic and elderly care doctors, lengths of stay on orthopaedic wards are shorter and more patients return home (Exhibit 14, overleaf).

54. There is insufficient evidence to support any single model of orthogeriatric liaison. Most professionals believe that the amount and quality of multidisciplinary assessment, care and therapy are the key factors, rather than any single element. There is even some evidence that specialist orthogeriatric units have higher costs and no better outcomes than ordinary wards where staff work effectively together to provide a high standard of care (Ref. 17).

55. If orthopaedic surgeons and their teams take a thorough comprehensive medical as well as multidisciplinary approach to rehabilitation and social care assessment, the need for input from elderly care doctors may be reduced. Some surgeons like to play a wide-ranging role, co-ordinating all aspects of the care of their patients. But others are primarily interested in surgical treatment, and prefer not to become involved with medical problems, rehabilitation and discharge planning. Under these circumstances, it is quite acceptable for them to pass on responsibility to others with access to a wider range of skills and resources although it is vital that all members of the team know where responsibility for each patient lies. At the Royal Infirmary, Edinburgh, physicians are involved right from the start, seeing patients even before the operation takes place, so that care is well integrated throughout their hospital stay (Case Study 3, overleaf).

56. The important thing is that arrangements should be clear and unambiguous so that somebody takes responsibility for all aspects of care and provides oversight, ensuring that all of the various stages in the care process fit together. The directorates of orthopaedics and elderly care share responsibility for ensuring that procedures, protocols, communication and liaison mechanisms have been established to ensure that this liaison happens in practice. This co-ordinated approach needs to continue throughout the process of rehabilitation, which necessarily involves many different professionals. The complexities of co-ordinating care are considered in the next chapter.

Exhibit 14
Effects of orthogeriatric liaison

Patients on wards with formal liaison are likely to be transferred more quickly...

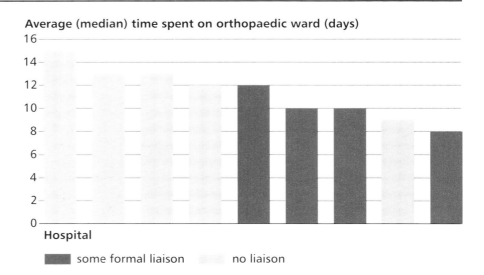

Average (median) time spent on orthopaedic ward (days)

...and are more likely to return home.

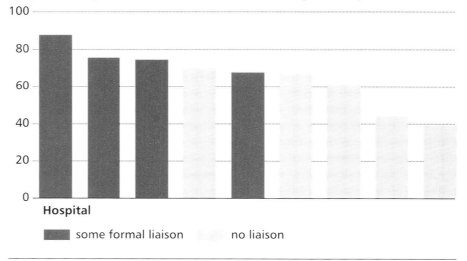

Proportion of patients admitted from home who go directly home

Source: 450 patient records at nine hospitals

Case Study 3
Well-established liaison

At the Royal Infirmary, Edinburgh, a staff grade physician in care of the elderly carries out a daily ward round in all trauma wards. This is backed up by a twice weekly multidisciplinary ward round which includes the elderly care consultant, orthopaedic house officer, nurses, physiotherapists, and occupational therapists.

The team aims to discover the medical and social problems of individual patients as soon as possible, so that post-operative care can be planned even before the operation. On one such ward round attended by the study team, most patients had other medical or social problems. One previously fit and active patient had a dependent relative, who needed to be looked after at home.

Evaluation suggests that there are few delays associated with surgery, transfer and discharge of hip fracture patients at this hospital.

Recommendations

The orthopaedic directorate, in consultation with managers and other theatre users, should:

1 allocate experienced staff to run trauma lists and supervise inexperienced junior doctors;

2 audit the number of operations performed by unsupervised junior doctors, and check that these operations are properly conducted;

3 ensure that there is sufficient operating time on day-time trauma lists for hip fracture patients;

4 audit the time to surgery for hip fracture patients, and investigate the reasons for delays;

5 establish standards, based on research, for withholding food and water from older patients prior to surgery; and

6 monitor cancelled operations and investigate the reasons.

The orthopaedic and elderly care directorates should:

7 ensure that specialist care is available for all elderly patients with fractured hips; and

8 jointly develop the necessary procedures, protocols, communication and liaison mechanisms to ensure that care is systematically planned and co-ordinated.

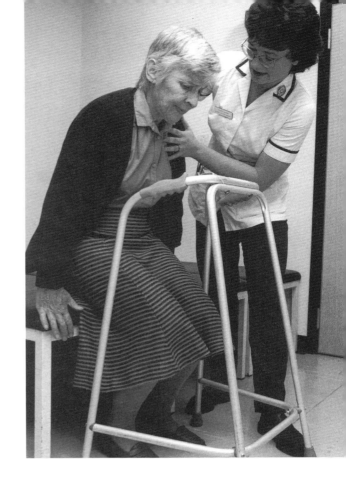

3 Rehabilitation and the Return Home

After surgery, most people want to return home, but many need a period of rehabilitation in order to do so. Few hospitals organise this aspect of care well, especially for people who need more time. Effective rehabilitation also requires good teamwork between the many professionals involved, further assessment and care planning to provide a positive approach, and suitable environments that allow people to recover at their own speed. Early discharge schemes which get people home with extensive support appear to be effective if well managed, although the amount of support must be sufficient.

Successful discharge from hospital depends on the early identification of people likely to need help, an early specification of a target date for discharge, and full assessment and planning of the support needed well in advance. Few hospitals adopt this approach and most need to improve their procedures.

57. After surgery and the resolution of any medical problems, most people want to return home, even though they may initially lack the confidence to do so. Regaining the ability to walk and cope with normal day-to-day activities, such as washing and dressing, are all important aspects of the rehabilitation process, helping people re-establish the skills they need when they leave hospital.

58. It is relatively straightforward to arrange a programme of rehabilitation for patients whose admission is planned in advance, such as hip replacement for arthritis. The timing of the operation is known beforehand, and patients are relatively healthy. Their social care needs and living arrangements can also be assessed before admission. For patients with a fractured hip who are admitted as emergencies to acute wards with an emphasis on short stay and quick turnover, however, this is not possible. Under these circumstances, arranging their rehabilitation and discharge planning is more difficult. It is, therefore, all the more important to have sound assessment procedures from the start.

Assessment and care planning

59. Rehabilitation requires careful assessment, planning and evaluation (Exhibit 15), which builds on the care planned and delivered when patients are first admitted (Chapter 1).

60. Thorough assessment increases professionals' knowledge of their patients, identifies problems, and provides a basis for evaluation. Standardising assessments increases their reliability and helps to ensure consistency. Assessment tools assist communication between professionals in the multidisciplinary team and with external agencies. They can also be used to monitor the progress of individuals, and therefore outcomes (Case Study 4, overleaf).

Exhibit 15
The rehabilitation cycle

Rehabilitation requires careful assessment, planning and evaluation.

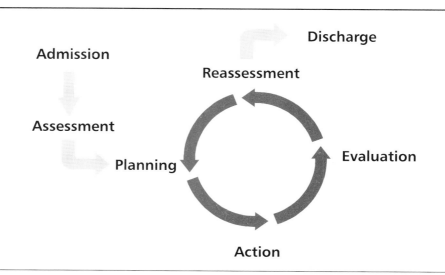

Source: Audit Commission

Case Study 4
Southampton

A multi-disciplinary team on acute elderly care wards in Southampton has incorporated standardised assessments in its practice. This has clinical benefits (as described above), but the team is also exploring ways of using assessment data to measure and improve the quality of service to patients.

The following information is collected about each patient:

Assessment tool	Timing
Barthel index and components	Admission Discharge Follow-up
Abbreviated mental test score	Admission Discharge Follow-up
Geriatric depression score	During inpatient care Follow-up
Philadelphia Geriatric Centre morale scale	During inpatient care Follow-up
Relatives' stress score	During inpatient care Follow-up

This gives a series of scores for outcomes, which are used to set future targets together with information about length of stay, mortality, re-admission rates and institutionalisation rates. Patients with particularly good or bad outcomes can also be identified, for peer review with casenote analysis.
(Ref.18)

61. A number of assessment tools in common use have already been mentioned. Some are used almost exclusively by nurses, while others are used by the whole multidisciplinary team. The most common of these are:

◆ pressure sore risk assessment;

◆ nutritional risk assessment;

◆ pain assessment;

◆ the Barthel Index, used to measure physical ability;

◆ the Geriatric Depression Score;

◆ the abbreviated mental test score, used to measure cognitive impairment; and

◆ the Philadelphia Geriatric Centre morale scale, used to measure perceived quality of life.

"One of the nurses told me 'you shouldn't be on so many pain killers', so the next time I was due for some, I wasn't in so much pain, so I said I could do without them. Then when I asked for them, the nurse said, 'Well, you refused them last time, it's your own fault.' I was given them, but I felt you couldn't win."

Controlling pain

62. The value of multidisciplinary assessment and planning is well illustrated in the management of pain. Pain is an almost inevitable side effect of a fracture and surgical repair. This pain, and that associated with other chronic disorders, can have a profound effect on a patient's ability to walk and willingness to participate in rehabilitation. Pain can also demotivate and demoralise. It can affect a patient's appetite, and lead to problems of incontinence and constipation since many patients find the lavatory or commode particularly uncomfortable following repair of a fracture.

63. Assessing and managing pain to avoid these problems requires good teamwork. Doctors are responsible for prescribing painkilling medication, while nurses are central to the assessment, management and evaluation of pain relief, since they spend most time with patients. In the past, pain control has often been based on rituals and routines, with standard drug regimes and subjective judgements. However, a variety of pain assessment tools now exist which aim to provide a more objective measure. Used consistently, these can be very effective in monitoring and evaluating pain relief.

64. A key variable in providing effective pain relief is continuity of care. This allows the patient to build up a relationship with a small group of nurses who become familiar with how that patient experiences pain. A plan of care can then be developed which includes comfortable positioning, strategies for movement, and effective analgesia.

65. The timing of pain relief is also important. Painkillers should be provided before procedures such as washing, turning and getting out of bed. Walking is particularly difficult if a patient is in pain or frightened of pain. Physiotherapists often complain that their ability to mobilise patients is compromised by analgesia given at the wrong time, either too early or too late, so that patients are in too much pain to participate willingly in rehabilitation.

Promoting mobility

66. One of the key elements of rehabilitation for hip fracture patients is to get them moving again as soon as possible after their operation. The Royal College of Physicians recommends only that plans for mobilisation, rehabilitation and discharge should be made within four days of operation, but already in some hospitals it is common for patients to be mobilised the day after surgery. Early mobilisation reduces the risk of complications and also promotes confidence (Refs. 4, 19).

67. At hospitals visited for this report practice was generally good, with most routinely encouraging patients to stand earlier than the Royal College of Physicians' recommendation. At two hospitals, however, no standard had been set (Exhibit 16, overleaf).

68. Immobility can have particularly serious consequences for older patients, causing pressure sores, deep vein thrombosis, and pneumonia, prolonging hospital stay, and reducing the likelihood of a patient returning to independent

Exhibit 16
Mobilisation after surgery

Practice was generally good. Seven out of nine hospitals routinely get patients back on their feet in the first two days after surgery.

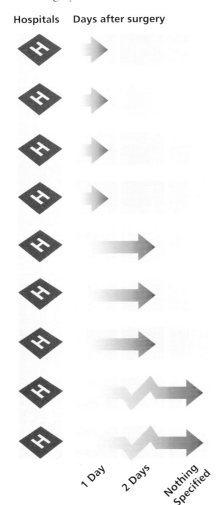

Hospitals   Days after surgery

1 Day   2 Days   Nothing Specified

Source: Audit Commission

living. An assessment of pre-operative mobility provides a baseline from which realistic and achievable goals can be set, and against which progress can be measured. It is also one of the best predictors of the patient's recovery. This assessment is an essential part of the multidisciplinary team's holistic plan of care for a patient, but it does not always happen in practice (Exhibit 8, page 17).

69. Once an assessment has been made and mobilisation goals set, a good ward environment encourages patients to move around. Some of the factors are obvious, but they may not exist on wards caring for elderly hip fracture patients:

- beds, chairs and toilets at the appropriate height for individual patients;
- non-slip floor surfaces;
- hand rails;
- good lighting;
- sign-posting of doorways, exits, toilets and bathrooms;
- easy access to glasses, hearing aids and walking aids; and
- easy access to personal belongings.

Encouraging independence

70. Apart from the specific interventions required to restore people's abilities, the multidisciplinary team can do a great deal to encourage independence and confidence by establishing the right environment. It has long been recognised that apparently simple factors such as clothing, the structure of the patient's day and the ward environment are crucial to a sense of dignity and autonomy.

71. On orthopaedic wards geared to short lengths of stay, patients may not be encouraged to dress at all, remaining instead in dressing gowns and slippers all day. And on some elderly care wards, patients still wear communal clothes, identified with a hospital property label, which are likely to be ill fitting or difficult to fasten. As well as the negative effect on dignity, this can make dressing and toileting difficult. Wearing ill-fitting shoes or slippers also makes walking more difficult and reduces confidence and morale.

72. None of the hospitals visited had washing machines close to orthopaedic or elderly care wards to enable patients to wear their own clothes. Patients on orthopaedic wards commonly wore night-clothes, even where they stayed on these wards throughout their hospital stay (often five weeks or more).

Case Study 5
Lings Bar House
Nottingham

This purpose-built. rehabilitation facility for elderly patients includes a laundry facility on site. Patients are encouraged to wear their own clothing which can be laundered and returned to them; the service is more efficient than using a hospital laundry service.

◆ Clothing is presentable and patients have a readily available supply;

◆ The turnaround time for garments is reduced and there is less risk of damage to clothing, as washing temperatures are more appropriate;

◆ The problem of lost clothing is reduced; and

◆ Patients' and relatives' satisfaction with the service is increased

"I was in there three weeks, they only made me walk three times. That is bad, they should have given me some exercises or therapy ... There was no instruction, and I was surprised because I couldn't walk."

73. Patients taking part in rehabilitation should also be encouraged to exercise control over their daily activities, from the time of meals and the choice of food, to the activities they undertake and the company they keep with other patients.

Teamwork

74. Teamwork is important when planning and delivering rehabilitation. Several groups of professionals are involved (Box C, overleaf).

75. These different professionals need to work together if patients are to gain the maximum benefit from rehabilitation. The Royal College of Physicians recommends that post-operative care should be carried out by a multidisciplinary team. Lines of communication should be clear and may involve weekly ward meetings, daily handovers, and joint working with patients, to ensure consistency and a patient-centred approach. Setting joint goals for rehabilitation helps to ensure that patients are neither over-protected, nor demoralised by over-ambitious expectations. Effective communication and planning help to ensure that patients continue their rehabilitation even when key members of the team are absent.

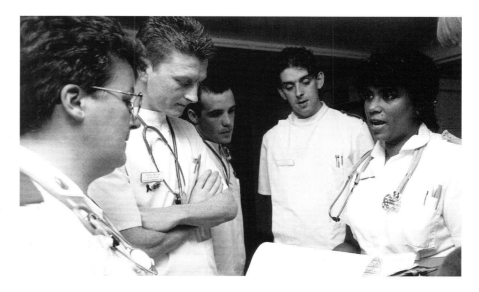

Box C
Roles of the main groups of
professionals involved

Consultant surgeons and physicians and their staff are responsible for diagnosing and treating surgical and medical problems and post-operative complications. They have a key role in stimulating the development of services, setting protocols and, through clinical audit, ensuring that these work smoothly in practice.

Physiotherapists are primarily concerned with mobility. They set goals for recovery, teaching patients to transfer in and out of bed and on and off chairs, to stand and to move around with walking aids. They design exercises to strengthen the muscles, improve balance and restore ability.

Occupational therapists help patients to cope with basic daily activities such as dressing, washing and preparing food and drink. They work with patients on the ward, and perhaps also in a specially designed kitchen, assessing the patient's abilities and devising ways to overcome problems. They may assess patients' home environments before discharge, and recommend aids and adaptations to help them cope at home.

Nurses are central to the rehabilitation process as, unlike the other professionals, they are always present on the ward. They continue the work started by therapists, making sure that patients carry out treatment plans and practise exercises. Good nursing itself furthers the rehabilitation process in a number of ways:
- tackling the problems of old age in a positive manner;
- encouraging patients to be independent; and
- reinforcing the patient's aim of returning home to independent living.

Social workers, or care assessors, plan and organise the social support people need when they leave hospital. They are also concerned with protecting the patient's rights and balancing the risks involved in discharge arrangements. They sometimes help to sort out financial matters.

76. For multidisciplinary working to be effective, someone should have overall responsibility for planning and reviewing the progress of each individual patient from day to day. While the consultant (either orthopaedic or elderly care) is responsible for patients in his or her care, the nurse – who has most contact with patients and carers – is well placed to co-ordinate the various professional groups on a day-to-day basis and liaise with the patient's family. Working as part of the multidisciplinary team, she or he should make sure that assessment, planning and communication between professionals, patients and their carers meet standards set by the directorates and by the hospital.

77. In spite of the clear advantages of a multidisciplinary approach to rehabilitation, it is not always achieved. The reasons for this identified at study hospitals included:
- poor referral practices;
- failures in communication;
- poor service organisation;
- inadequate staffing levels; and
- problems in organising aids and appliances.

Referrals

78. Some therapists, especially occupational therapists, will only see patients after they have been referred by doctors or nurses. This means that patients are likely to wait longer to be seen, with some who could benefit not being referred at all. A better service is provided where therapists visit trauma wards daily so that they know of all patients admitted or operated on during the previous 24 hours, enabling contact to be made more quickly, and minimising the danger of patients being 'missed'.

Communication

79. Communication between professionals is not always effective. Surgeons may leave therapists to plan treatment and nurses to make discharge arrangements. And although they do not work in total isolation, the different professionals involved rarely come together to discuss plans and progress except during ward rounds (none did so regularly at the nine hospitals visited). Most communication between staff is informal, and informality, combined with dispersed responsibility, can lead to poor communication. Therapists invariably keep their own notes, and if they fail to write in medical or nursing notes, other team members may not keep up to date with plans and progress.

Service organisation

80. The organisation of services may also cause problems. Therapists may be attached to specialties, or more narrowly to wards or consultants. In one hospital studied, physiotherapists are linked to consultants with patients on a number of different wards. They find it very difficult to organise sufficient time with nurses, occupational therapists and social workers on each ward. A ward-based service means that there are less likely to be gaps in the service; it is easier to keep up to date with new admissions, and to get to know the other professionals working on the ward. Six out of the nine hospitals studied allocated therapists to wards.

Staffing levels

81. Posts for therapy staff are frequently unfilled, particularly occupational therapists. In one large acute hospital studied, there were only 1.5 occupational therapists to cover all wards. The senior therapist has resorted to producing written information for hip fracture patients which she distributes even if she is unable to spend any time with them. Nurses are responsible for the tasks normally undertaken by occupational therapists, but home visits are difficult to arrange and sometimes take place after the patient has been discharged. Hospitals must ensure they have sufficient staff to fulfil their responsibilities.

Aids and adaptations

82. Finally, it may be difficult to obtain aids and adaptations required by patients on discharge. Some services have organised on-site stores for small items, and this can help to prevent delays. It is often easier to obtain aids where district stores are run jointly by health and social services.

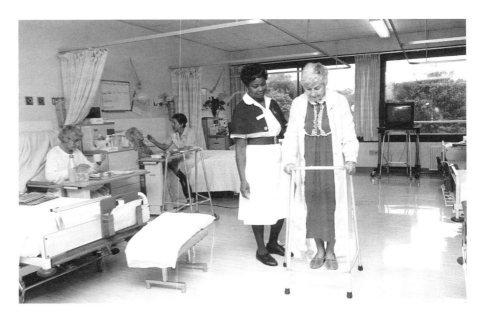

Providing the right environment

83. For hip fracture patients, rehabilitation may happen in a number of different places. The most common options include:

- orthopaedic wards, where patients stay until they leave hospital;
- specialist orthogeriatric units;
- general elderly rehabilitation wards; and
- early supported discharge or hospital-at-home schemes.

84. Again, the particular location is less important than the ability to gear the content of the rehabilitation process to the needs of individual patients. It is rare, however, for services to be designed to meet the whole range of needs (Exhibit 17). Sometimes there is a scheme for those who are likely to recover quickly; in other cases, there is an option for the slow stream rehabilitation of patients who would otherwise 'block' orthopaedic beds.

Orthopaedic wards

85. Rehabilitation always starts on orthopaedic wards, and should begin as soon as possible after the operation to repair the fracture. Some of the more able patients may be fit enough to go home unaided after just a week or two, requiring no additional provision; but many people take longer to regain their confidence. For such people, a busy orthopaedic ward is not the best place to recover, and a variety of alternatives are offered by different hospitals.

Specialist orthogeriatric units

86. Some hospitals have established special units for elderly orthopaedic patients, with care provided by both orthopaedic surgeons and elderly care doctors. These offer the benefits of all good orthogeriatric liaison, but there is some evidence that the additional costs produce outcomes that are no better than cheaper alternatives.

General elderly rehabilitation wards

87. At many hospitals, patients may be transferred to a rehabilitation ward for older patients recovering from a range of problems including fractures, surgical operations and strokes. The reason behind the transfer is not always the rehabilitation care available; in one hospital, the decision to move patients is made each morning by nurses on the surgical ward – patients are moved only if that ward has a shortage of beds. If there is no demand patients stay, whether rehabilitation beds are available or not. Patients and carers may be given very little, if any, notice of transfers.

"[on the day of transfer] a young nurse came and said how would I like to move? I didn't realise she meant to [the rehabilitation hospital]."

Exhibit 17
Rehabilitation schemes for elderly orthopaedic patients

Few hospitals provide something for everyone.

Hospitals	Fast stream	Slow stream
H	Jointly funded social services and community health services residential rehabilitation facility	
H	Rehabilitation unit used primarily for joint replacement patients	Orthogeriatric unit with shared care between orthopaedics and care of the elderly
H	Hospital at home	
H		
H	Beds on orthopaedic ward where patients are under elderly care physicians	
H	Orthogeriatric beds	
H	Community health services rehabilitation facility for patients expected to return home quickly	
H		
H		

where nothing is shown, rehabilitation takes place on orthopaedic wards

where nothing is shown, orthopaedic surgeons depend on formal referral to care of the elderly doctors for patients who need longer term care.

Source: Audit Commission

Residential and nursing homes

88. As the community care arrangements become established, new options for rehabilitation are emerging (Case Studies 6 and 7). The aim behind these is often to allow time for elderly people to regain their abilities and their confidence after a crisis such as a fractured hip. This may be sufficient to avoid the need for a move to residential or nursing home care, increasing the independence of the patient and reducing the long-term cost of care.

89. The distinguishing elements of these schemes are that active therapy and rehabilitation are available, and that the stay is carefully planned. It is important to distinguish between rehabilitation and convalescence facilities. In convalescence, there is no active programme to restore patients' abilities and independence. The value of traditional convalescence beds is highly questionable. The longer patients are kept inactive and away from their usual environment, the more difficult it is for them to cope when they eventually return. The only benefit of convalescent beds is as a means of emptying acute orthopaedic beds. Patients gain very little.

Early supported discharge

90. Rehabilitation need not be offered in hospital, and there can be real advantages in using community settings for patients who are well enough. Only home-based rehabilitation services, such as hospital-at-home or early discharge schemes, offer patients the opportunity to learn how to cope in their usual surroundings. This is important; there is a huge difference between the hospital environment, with even floors, wide corridors and specially designed, spacious kitchens, and people's own homes with obstacles and limited space. Patients and carers are very aware of the practical problems.

Case Study 6 **Community Assessment, Rehabilitation and Treatment Project** **Cornwall**	The teams were designed to offer skilled multidisciplinary assessments of health and social care needs under the NHS and Community Care Act, particularly for people verging on the threshold of institutional care. Two teams were established, consisting of physiotherapy and occupational therapy staff, and a specialist support nurse, with referral to a consultant elderly care physician as needed. Significant improvements in patients' Barthel scores were observed compared with a control group, and there were fewer admissions to institutional care.
Case Study 7 **Rehabilitation from a residential home base** **Devon, Dorset, Hampshire**	Three former residential homes offer short-term rehabilitation for users who are determined to return to their own homes, but who need time and support to regain their skills and confidence. The setting is residential, but physiotherapy and occupational therapy are key parts of the care provided. Admissions are for a set period (usually up to six weeks), and a target date for going home is identified at the outset.

"One of the things they don't tell you about is the difference between the wide open spaces of the hospital and your cramped home."

91. A properly resourced early discharge scheme, offered as a choice to patients, is one way of making sure that rehabilitation is tailored to individual needs. It also helps to ensure a smooth handover between hospital and community staff, improving working relationships in the process. It may help to avoid discharges to residential or nursing homes which, even as temporary arrangements, can lead to long term dependency.

92. Two of the study hospitals had orthopaedic hospital-at-home schemes, but only one included hip fracture patients. The study team also visited the Peterborough hospital-at-home scheme, the longest running in the country (Case Study 8), and the Edinburgh early supported discharge service (Case Study 9).

93. All hospitals visited during the study without hospital-at-home schemes are currently considering establishing them. This is partly to reduce lengths of stay in hospital, and partly because purchasers and providers are keen to shift the balance of care in favour of the community. Initial costings suggest that hospital-at-home schemes cost less than inpatient care for hip fracture patients (Ref. 20), but the resource implications should be considered carefully when

---

Case Study 8
Peterborough 'hospital-at-home' scheme

The service is district-wide and has been running for 17 years. Responsibility for medical care lies with the patient's GP, who has immediate access to a hospital bed if there are problems.

For hip fracture patients, hospital-at-home offers:
◆ discharge soon after surgery;
◆ assessment by a district nurse;
◆ support according to the patient's needs – nursing care may initially be available 24 hours a day;
◆ physiotherapy;
◆ occupational therapy; and
◆ patient aides to provide help and support.

Case Study 9
Edinburgh early supported discharge

The Royal Infirmary, Edinburgh, has established an early supported discharge scheme for fitter hip fracture patients. The aim is to enable them to be discharged directly home from acute orthopaedic care, with rehabilitation and reliable post-discharge support.

A liaison occupational therapist and a liaison sister have been appointed to work with the orthopaedic nursing and rehabilitation staff and an elderly care doctor. The team promotes and monitors early rehabilitation, carries out pre-discharge assessment and home visits, liaises with community health and social services, and monitors progress after the patient has gone home.

The proportion of hip fracture patients going straight home from acute care has risen, and satisfaction is high among patients, their carers, GPs and community health and social services staff. Economic evaluation has shown that the scheme has brought considerable savings by reducing lengths of stay.

new schemes are being set up. Hospital-at-home schemes must have sufficient resources to work properly.

Going home

94. Discharge home is the final stage of the patient's hospital stay, and it should be the culmination of all that has gone before rather than an afterthought. All care should be directed towards a successful transfer. If the other aspects of care, from admission, through acute care to rehabilitation, are planned properly, then good discharge will follow on as a natural consequence. If, on the other hand, any part of this process is missed or skimped, the consequences are likely to emerge around discharge. The process can be likened to a relay race, with every stage equally important if success is to be the end result.

95. The Department of Health has issued guidance over the years in the form of circulars in 1989 (Ref. 21) and a hospital discharge workbook in 1994 (Ref. 22). More recently, the Department has issued guidance requiring the NHS to clarify its responsibilities for continuing health care needs (Ref. 23), fully consulting and involving local authorities, GPs, users, carers and others. The result should be clearer definitions of when people are ready for discharge.

96. In practice, various steps are needed to integrate discharge planning with earlier stages, involving patients and their carers fully and keeping them informed at each stage:

- identification of people who are likely to need help after discharge, and the type and extent of help they are likely to need;
- early specification of a likely target date for discharge, and involvement of all who need to plan care after discharge; and
- full assessment of the situation as the target date approaches (including home visits where appropriate), and planning of support during and after discharge;
- organisation of the support required.

Identification

97. Identifying who is likely to need help can start right at the very beginning – possibly in A&E but certainly during the initial assessment on the ward. The detailed nature of the help needed cannot be defined at the start, because the outcome of the operation and other treatment, and response to the rehabilitation programme, are not yet known, and both profoundly affect the degree of support needed. But people living on their own with limited mobility or with some confusion can be identified if the assessment process is effective. Such information needs to be recorded clearly on the notes and even included in some form of monitoring system, so that all are aware of a likely need for future action.

Specifying a target date for discharge

98. Discharge from hospital should be part of the planning process for rehabilitation once the operation is over – even though the date is likely to be vague to start with. Assigning people to a 'fast stream' and 'slow stream' is a first step in this process; as rehabilitation progresses, it is possible to be more specific about a likely date. Once such a date has been specified, it should be recorded in the notes and those responsible for organising post-discharge care alerted.

Assessment and planning

99. This can start in good time before the target date, allowing post-discharge care to be planned as a continuation of the rehabilitation programme rather than as a provision hastily put in place to clear a bed. Where there is a hospital-at-home or early discharge scheme, this continuation tends to take place naturally, as these schemes are short term and linked to what has gone before. Where there is no such scheme, the danger is that discharge breaks the pattern of support, undermining the rehabilitation process. This is especially so if discharge planning does not take account of the rehabilitation programme, and may lead to care that is inappropriate, such as unnecessary admission to a residential or nursing home in spite of progress made through rehabilitation. Where the rehabilitation is complete there is no such problem, but many people – especially those on the 'slow stream' – continue to need rehabilitation for a long time.

Organisation of support

100. Support needs to be effective so that people do not go home to an empty house and empty larder in spite of well-laid plans.

101. As part of this study, patient records were examined for evidence of discharge planning. The results were poor at all hospitals (Exhibit 18, overleaf).

"I was discharged with no aftercare, no appointment for physio ... I was just dropped by the ambulance and that was it ... I found it very difficult."

102. Patients' views of discharge were often negative. Many said they were given conflicting information, and carers were critical of the lack of planning and consultation. Written information is rarely provided. At five hospitals, social care assessors said that written information about services is available for patients, but at only one is it used routinely.

103. Carers were critical of the lack of active discharge planning and consultation with them.

Exhibit 18
Discharge planning documentation

Discharge planning is poorly recorded in patient records.

■ Yes
▢ No

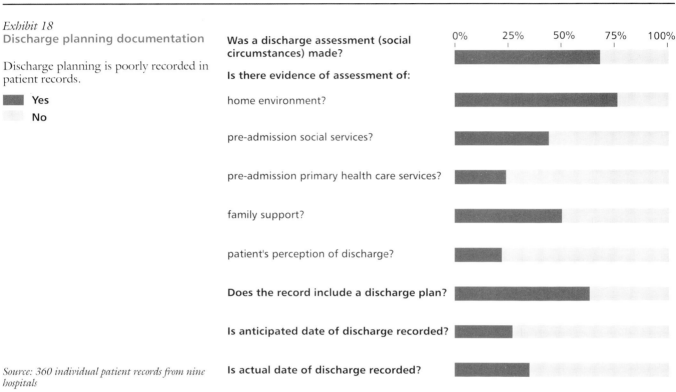

Source: 360 individual patient records from nine hospitals

"My husband felt they were pushing all the time to get her out whether she was well or not ... we had to have the toilet [being installed downstairs] ready for her."

104. Factors which contributed to this poor performance included:

◆ little awareness of the hospital discharge policy. Ward sisters were often unable to provide a copy of the policy, or to give a clear description of its contents;

◆ few formal planning meetings. Multi-disciplinary meetings may only take place during ward rounds, which are often inconvenient for staff based elsewhere, such as social workers or therapists. Some wards do not have meetings at all;

◆ a lack of training for nurses and social workers. Most hospitals rely on cascade training for nurses, with little or no direct training. Although most social workers received some training when community care responsibilities were introduced, many said the focus was on how to complete forms; and

◆ poor monitoring of discharge, with unclear responsibilities and poor information. Re-admissions are rarely monitored.

Discharge policy

105. Hospitals have been required since 1989 to establish and set out clear procedures for discharge and make these known to staff. All hospitals visited had policies, but staff rarely referred to them. In some hospitals, social workers were unfamiliar with the hospital discharge policy, and ward staff in turn were unfamiliar with the standards and triggers for referral to social services. Social workers did not routinely attend ward round meetings on orthopaedic wards at any of the hospitals visited during the study, although most did attend multidisciplinary meetings on elderly care wards.

106. Perhaps more significantly, there appeared to be few attempts to estimate the resource consequences of hospital policies. Social services assessors reported difficulties in arranging complex care packages for hospital patients because of a shortage of resources. The requirements to clarify NHS responsibilities for meeting continuing health care needs (Ref. 23) should start to quantify some of these needs and resource requirements, confronting policymakers with the financial consequences of current arrangements.

107. This lack of common understanding causes major problems in planning rehabilitation and discharge. Hospital staff are under constant pressure to discharge patients; the decision to discharge may be made during a ward round and the patient is expected to go home the same day. Social services assessors, on the other hand, are under pressure to tailor individual care packages and to remain within limited budgets. This takes time.

108. These working practices are incompatible: in the worst cases, ward staff do not make a referral to social services until a patient is ready to go home. Social services staff do not have time to do their job properly, and conflict results. A more co-operative approach is needed. Developing a shared understanding of the goals and tasks of both parties requires careful planning (Case Study 10)

Case Study 10
Joint working between health and social services

At North Tyneside Trust, a discharge policy was agreed by a working group made up of:

- general managers from each directorate, responsible for liaising with doctors and other professional groups;
- ward nurses;
- district nurses;
- the community development manager;
- social services manager and hospital social workers;
- a community health council representative; and
- a GP.

A simple 'traffic light' system is used on all wards to identify those who need referral to social services. Joint training takes place for ward sisters, district nurses and social workers.

The working group is developing discharge standards and shared documentation.

Formal planning meetings

109. Successful discharge planning needs to bring together professionals from hospital, community health and social services. The difficulty of achieving this is increased when patients are admitted from outside the hospital's normal catchment area, perhaps because they have sustained a fracture while on holiday.

110. Discharge liaison nurses often provide a link between hospital and community, attending discharge planning meetings and getting to know the needs of individual patients. However, this role can introduce its own problems. A single discharge liaison nurse may be unable to cover a whole hospital effectively; in one study hospital the discharge liaison nurse works mainly on elderly care wards, and only visits the orthopaedic wards if invited.

111. In addition, the presence of a discharge liaison nurse may mean that ward nurses do not take responsibility for discharge planning and fail to learn about local services. A more useful role for liaison nurses would be to establish frameworks for liaison between services, and help ward and community staff to develop their own arrangements.

112. Such frameworks are essential if staff are to work together. No single model is likely to be successful and each locality must develop its own method of working, perhaps with regular team meetings. The main point is that there should be a recognition that some formal arrangement is required and that it is made to work.

- **Training** should ensure that all the professionals involved know the procedures and how to apply them. Joint training between health and social services staff are to be preferred if at all possible.

- **Monitoring** is needed to ensure that discharge is effective. *The Hospital Discharge Workbook* (Ref. 23) proposes a list of possible performance indicators which hospitals can use.

113. Hospital discharge should be seen as a way of bringing all other actions within the hospital to a satisfactory conclusion, but appears at present to be poorly co-ordinated in some hospitals. Priority should be given not simply to passing the patient on to the next stage but to ensuring that every stage of the care process contributes to a successful conclusion.

'Priority should be given not simply to passing the patient on to the next stage but to ensuring that every stage of the care process contributes to a successful conclusion.'

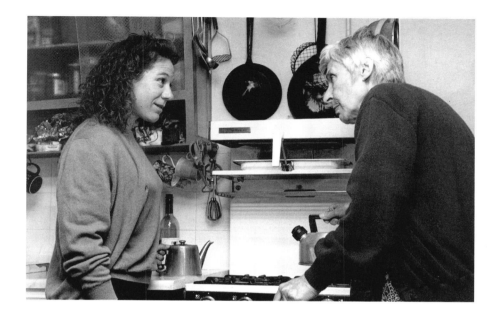

Recommendations

Clinicians should work together to establish:

1   standard assessment procedures for patients who have fractured a hip, using validated assessment tools. These should be used as a basis for planning and evaluating care; and

2   target times for mobilising patients after their operations, together with arrangements for maximising their mobility and independence while in hospital.

Professionals and managers should:

3   work together to develop a formal multidisciplinary team approach, with clear lines of communication and joint goals for patients. A named individual (probably a primary nurse) should take overall responsibility for planning and reviewing the progress of each individual patient from day to day, keeping them and their carers fully informed of developments at all stages.

Therapists should:

4   visit trauma wards daily to see all patients admitted or operated on during the previous 24 hours.

Commissioners and trusts should:

5   ensure that they provide rehabilitation options for the whole range of needs, from those who are likely to recover quickly to those who will take much longer and require a good deal of support; and

6 ensure that trusts have comprehensive arrangements in place for:

- identification of people who are likely to need help after discharge, and the type and extent of help they are likely to need,
- early specification of a likely target date for discharge, and involvement of all who need to plan care,
- full assessment as the target date approaches (including home visits where appropriate),
- organisation of the support required, and
- ensuring that patients and their relatives are fully involved throughout the process;
- monitoring patients' progress towards discharge and the causes for delays.

Health and social services agencies must:

7 work together to develop a shared understanding of the roles and responsibilities of each in the discharge process.

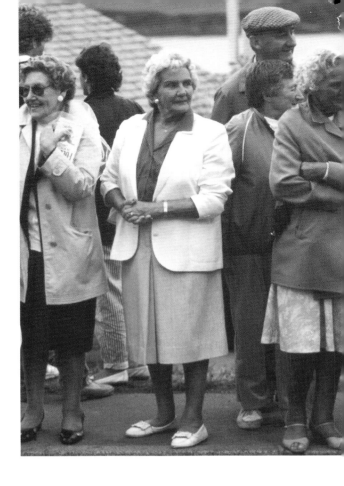

For care to be effective, each element must be provided as part of a co-ordinated package supervised by a named person. Purchasers could take a lead by specifying contracts for care by condition, incorporating the good practice described in this report.

The lessons learned from this study can be applied to other complex conditions requiring co-ordinated care from different professionals and agencies. As the population ages, better management of the care of elderly people is vital if the health service is to meet the challenges facing it.

4 Wider Lessons

114. If care is to be effective, each of the stages reported in the previous three chapters must be well managed. But, in addition, the overall process of care needs attention. The East Anglian audit referred to in the Introduction (Ref. 4) concluded that it was the total package of care rather than any single factor that improved outcomes. And the findings reported in Chapter 2 indicated that people's chances of going back to their own homes after their stay in hospital were enhanced by effective joint working between care of the elderly doctors and orthopaedic surgeons. Both rehabilitation and discharge are easier to plan if good assessments are available from the start.

115. All of these considerations point to the need for effective co-ordination. Many patients who fracture their hips have multiple problems and receive care from a number of professionals in a number of different locations. And yet, all too often, no one is clearly placed to provide this co-ordination, either from within the hospital or from the purchaser. The result is care that is fragmented and disjointed, with adverse effects on the outcomes for patients. What is needed is someone to take overall responsibility, supported by appropriate tools to help co-ordination proceed smoothly.

The purchaser

116. Purchasers are clearly responsible for ensuring that care is provided that meets the needs of people who have fractured their hips. But few are in a position to discharge this responsibility. Most purchasing in health authorities is undertaken through block contracts which specify the service required, usually in terms of a specialty, such as orthopaedic care or accident and emergency services. Such contracts mirror the fragmentation of treatment within hospitals described in this report.

117. To tackle the problems described, purchasers would need to start commissioning care by condition rather than by service – purchasing care for people who fracture their hips, for example. Contracts set in this way would look very different from traditional contracts and could start to specify some of the good practice described in this report (Box D, overleaf). In theory, fundholders could take this more patient-oriented approach, although, unless they are part of the new experimental group of 'total' fundholders, they are not yet responsible for purchasing emergency care.

118. The value of multi-centre clinical audits has been shown in East Anglia (Ref. 4), Scotland (Ref. 25) and Sweden (Ref. 26), all of which have highlighted significant differences between hospitals in the care provided and the outcomes for patients who have fractured a hip. This condition is particularly suitable for clinical audit, since it is significant in terms of the numbers of people affected and the cost of treating them, it is readily identifiable as a distinct condition, and research has identified many of the factors which are associated with a successful outcome. Purchasers should therefore consider including a requirement for regular clinical audit within their contracts for hip fracture services. The proportion of patients returning home is a key indicator of success.

Box D
A contract for purchasing care for people who have fractured their hips might include:

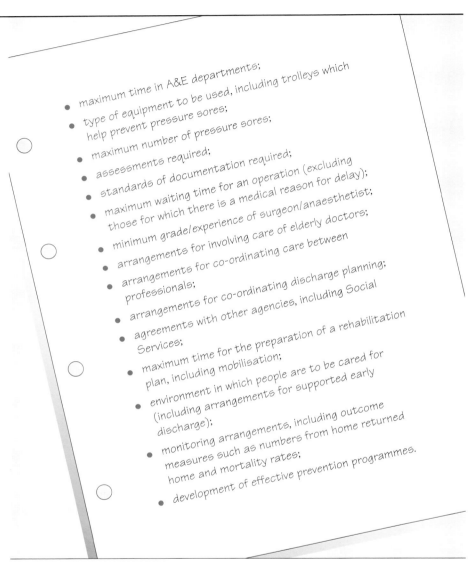

- maximum time in A&E departments;
- type of equipment to be used, including trolleys which help prevent pressure sores;
- maximum number of pressure sores;
- assessments required;
- standards of documentation required;
- maximum waiting time for an operation (excluding those for which there is a medical reason for delay);
- minimum grade/experience of surgeon/anaesthetist;
- arrangements for involving care of elderly doctors;
- arrangements for co-ordinating care between professionals;
- arrangements for co-ordinating discharge planning;
- agreements with other agencies, including Social Services;
- maximum time for the preparation of a rehabilitation plan, including mobilisation;
- environment in which people are to be cared for (including arrangements for supported early discharge);
- monitoring arrangements, including outcome measures such as numbers from home returned home and mortality rates;
- development of effective prevention programmes.

Hospitals providing care

119. This agenda must be worked out carefully with hospitals, with targets set by purchasers and costs worked out by providers (to provide equipment, meet targets, etc). Hospitals will need to have good internal procedures that specify both who is responsible for co-ordinating care, and systems for recording progress using the casenotes as the central record and method of communication between professionals. In many situations, doctors will take the lead but others such as nurses are also well placed to act as key workers for progressing care (by acting as 'named nurse', for example).

Services for older people in general

'Multiple medical and social problems are common to many older people, and their care requires a comprehensive approach which addresses all of their problems.'

120. Many elderly people undergo a similar pattern of care in hospital, with admission through A&E, treatment requiring co-ordinated care from different doctors, rehabilitation and discharge home requiring the involvement of different professionals and agencies, often over an extended period of time. Equally, the lessons learned from this study of a group of hip fracture patients can be applied more widely:

◆ time in A&E needs to be managed carefully to ensure that frail, elderly people do not spend considerable amounts of time waiting. A separate report to be published early in 1996 considers the management of A&E departments in more detail and provides guidance on how to reduce and contain waiting times;

◆ full assessments are needed for all elderly people admitted to hospital. Multiple medical and social problems are common to many older people, and their care requires a comprehensive approach which addresses all of their problems. Conditions such as pressure sores are not restricted to hip fracture patients;

◆ the involvement of physicians specialising in the care of the elderly is desirable for many older people who have some specific condition which brings them onto general wards. Working arrangements which involve physicians specialising in the care of the elderly are needed throughout the hospital;

◆ the need for a programme of rehabilitation is common to most older people who have suffered a major illness, and this programme needs to have all of the characteristics described in this report; and

◆ the need for well-managed arrangements for discharging people from hospital is widely recognised. Again, the principles described in this report and in Department of Health guidance are not restricted to hip fracture patients.

121. All of this care requires co-ordinating, just as it does for hip fracture patients. Those co-ordinating the care of people with mental health problems face a similarly complex task and are addressing it by adopting the Care Programme Approach (CPA) which specifies how the required co-ordination is to be achieved. The aim of the CPA is to ensure that:

◆ the patient's health and social care needs are systematically assessed;

◆ a care plan to meet these needs is agreed;

◆ a key worker is nominated to co-ordinate the implementation of the plan; and

◆ the patient's progress is regularly reviewed.

122. Following the CPA does not mean involving the whole multidisciplinary team in the care of each patient. If a patient has less complex needs, the assessment and care planning process will be relatively straightforward. Full multidisciplinary care and treatment should be reserved for those with the most complex needs. However, to ensure that no one falls through the net, everyone should receive a comprehensive assessment. A similar approach for elderly patients with complex conditions would have significant benefits in ensuring that care is planned and delivered as effectively as possible.

Exhibit 19
The changes projected for the population of older people (1992 – 2031)

The number of people aged 65 and over is projected to increase by 60 per cent by 2031.

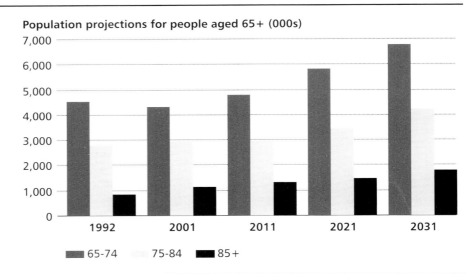

Population projections for people aged 65+ (000s)

Legend: 65-74 | 75-84 | 85+

Source: Office of Population Censuses and Surveys

123. The complex needs of elderly patients cannot be marginalised and left to specialist services, since older people are already major users of mainstream health and social services. People over 65 account for 60 per cent of all days spent in hospital in the four largest specialties (general medicine, general surgery, trauma and orthopaedics and urology). They account for over half the expenditure on primary care services and two-fifths of the expenditure on personal social services.

124. The demand for care will grow for a number of reasons. The number of people in the UK aged 65 and over is projected to increase by 60 per cent over the next 35 years, from about 8 million to almost 13 million. Over the same period, the number of 'very elderly' people aged 85 and over will more than double, from just under one million to almost two million (Exhibit 19).

125. At the same time, support from other sources is declining. The demographic shift means that the growing elderly population will be supported by proportionately fewer people of working age. And changing social patterns mean that an increasing proportion of women work outside the home, while smaller families are less able to take care of an older relative.

126. Taken together, these changes mean that pressure on health and social services is likely to grow significantly, increasing the need to use resources as effectively as possible. To do this, health services must aim to keep people fully independent for as long as possible. Anything less reduces their quality of life and increases the cost of caring for them.

Last word to the patients

127. Throughout this report the views of the patients themselves have been reported. Throughout it has been clear that they are not often kept informed of what is going on. Most of the quotes from the College of Health study are connected in one way or another with communication problems. Only one hospital visited had written information for hip fracture patients, although it was common for those undergoing hip replacement operations.

128. Perhaps more importantly, patients' comments suggested that they did not feel sufficiently involved in decisions about their care; they did not know what decisions had been taken, or why, in relation to key issues such as rehabilitation, discharge and support at home. The involvement of patients and their carers and relatives is crucial if they are to return home safely and successfully.

'The involvement of patients and their carers and relatives is crucial if they are to return home safely and successfully.'

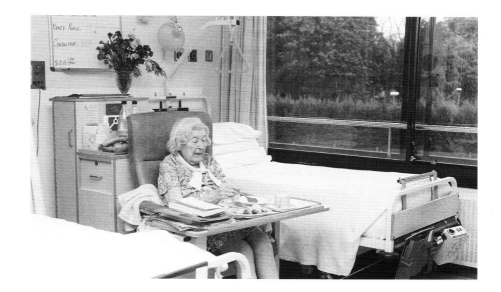

Getting It Right

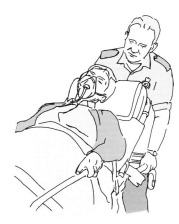

Mrs Green fell and fractured her hip. She was taken to hospital by ambulance, and on arrival in the A&E Department she was assessed by a nurse. The assessment considered her pressure sore risk and pain, and also reviewed her past medical history. The nurse found that Mrs Green was at high risk of pressure sores, so she transferred her to a pressure-relieving surface to reduce the risk. She also discovered that Mrs Green had had a stroke three years earlier, which meant that she walked with a stick before her fall.

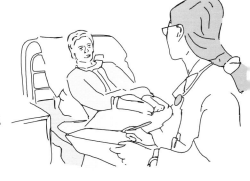

The hospital had a protocol for managing elderly patients with fractured hips. Mrs Green was quickly seen by a doctor, given painkillers and treated as a priority for x-ray. Within 30 minutes her x-ray had been reviewed by the radiologist and A&E doctors, the fracture had been confirmed, and the orthopaedic SHO on call had agreed to admit her.

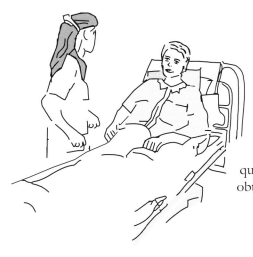

On the ward, information from her A&E assessment was transferred with her. She was immediately placed on a pressure-relieving bed, and when she was comfortable a nurse carried out a full assessment. This covered nutrition, pain, continence, mental state, previous mobility and social circumstances. In response to questions, Mrs Green told the nurse that she had always lived independently and that she wanted to return home as soon as possible. She was also quickly assessed by the orthopaedic SHO who reassured her and obtained her consent for an operation.

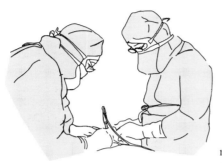

The operation to fix Mrs Green's fracture was carried out at the end of the regular trauma list that afternoon, by an experienced orthopaedic surgeon. When she returned to the ward her pain was assessed and painkilling drugs were prescribed to make her comfortable. When she awoke next morning she was relatively comfortable, and when the multidisciplinary team made its ward round, plans were made to get her back on her feet. The team planned input from physiotherapists and occupational therapists, and made initial plans for Mrs Green to be discharged home with intensive support from the local hospital-at-home scheme the following week.

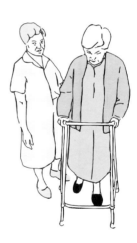

During her stay on the orthopaedic ward, Mrs Green had intensive physiotherapy, and learned to get in and out of bed and a chair and to walk again using a Zimmer frame. The occupational therapist assessed her ability to cope at home during a home visit, and arranged for a raised toilet seat to be fitted before Mrs Green's discharge.

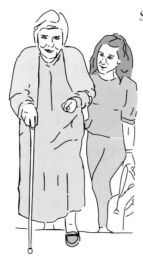

She was discharged as planned, with visits from the district nurse three times a day for the first four days. The physiotherapist also continued to visit for the first two weeks, to ensure that Mrs Green was continuing to develop her ability to move about her home and to help solve any problems. Two weeks after discharge, Mrs Green had progressed from a Zimmer frame to a pair of walking sticks. The district nurse was visiting every four days, and Mrs Green was continuing to improve.

Appendix 1: The Advisory Group

Thanks are due for the advice and guidance of the following people, who were members of the external advisory group to the project:

Roger Beech	Senior Research Fellow, Department of Public Health, St. Thomas's Hospital
Pearl Brown	Chief Executive, Riverside Community Healthcare NHS Trust
Tony Christopher	Audit Commissioner
Anna Culot	Association of Chartered Physiotherapists representative, with a special interest in elderly people
Edward Dickinson	Royal College of Physicians Research Unit
Anne Gaskell	College of Occupational Therapists representative
Chris Joyce	Department of Health
Dr David Kennie	Consultant Physician in Geriatric Medicine, Stirling Royal Infirmary
John Langan	Chief Executive, Kingston Hospital NHS Trust
Mr Alan Lettin	President, British Orthopaedics Association
Mr Raymond Newman	Orthopaedic Surgeon, Harrogate District Hospital
Professor Ian Philp	Northern General Hospital, Sheffield
Mr Glyn Prior	Orthopaedic Surgeon, Peterborough District Hospital
Eileen Shepherd	Independent Nursing Consultant; former Ward Sister, Care of the Elderly Department, Queen's Medical Centre, Nottingham
Neil Walker	Director of Social Services, London Borough of Barking & Dagenham
Jane Whelan	Age Concern, England
Simon Williams	Basingstoke & North Hants Health Authority

Appendix 2: Royal College of Physicians' Recommendations

Managers and clinicians should:

- allocate responsibility for reviewing services, producing a strategy and monitoring standards of care and outcome;
- review mortality and morbidity annually;
- undertake studies to investigate different management strategies;
- ensure that patients spend no more than one hour in A&E;
- include assessment of co-existing medical problems, mental function and social circumstances into pre-operative planning;
- begin discharge planning at the assessment stage;
- ensure operations are carried out within 24 hours by senior staff;
- make plans for mobilisation, rehabilitation and discharge/transfer within four days of the operation;
- ensure close working relationships between orthopaedic surgeons and geriatricians;
- make available experienced nurses, physiotherapy and occupational therapy services; and
- provide a means of liaison with community services and carers.

References

1. Department of Public Health Medicine, *Effective Healthcare Bulletin No. 1: Screening for Osteoporosis to Prevent Fractures,* University of Leeds, 1991

2. National Osteoporosis Society, *Priorities for Prevention – Osteoporosis: A Decision-Making Document for Diagnosis and Prevention,* NOS, 1995

3. W J Boyce and M P Vessey, 'Rising incidence of fracture of the proximal femur', *The Lancet,* i, 1985, pp150-1

4. C J Todd et al, 'Differences in mortality after fracture of hip: The East Anglian audit', *British Medical Journal,* Vol. 310, 1995, pp904-8

5. Royal College of Physicians, *Fractured Neck of Femur: Prevention and Management,* RCP, 1989

6. The British Geriatrics Society, the Royal College of Psychiatrists and the Royal College of Nursing, *Improving the Care of Elderly People in Hospital,* RCN, 1987

7. RCN Standards of Care Project, *Standards of Care in Orthopaedic Nursing* (1990) and *Nursing Older People* (1991), RCN

8. Royal College of Physicians of London and British Geriatrics Society, *Standardised Assessment Scales for Elderly People: A Report of Joint Workshops of the Research Unit of the Royal College of Physicians and the British Geriatrics Society,* 1992

9. Department of Health, *Pressure Sores: A Key Quality Indicator -A Guide for NHS Purchasers and Providers,* DoH, 1995

10. NHS Executive, VFM Update Issue No. 12, *Pressure Sores: A Preventable Problem,* DoH, 1994

11. M J Parker, G A Prior, J W Myles, 'The value of a special surgical team in preventing complications in the treatment of hip fractures', *International Orthopaedics* (SICOT), Vol. 18, pp184-8

12. J V Perez, D J Warwick, C P Case, G C Bannister, 'Death after proximal femoral fracture – an autopsy study', *Injury,* Vol. 26, 1995, pp237-40

13. British Orthopaedics Association, *The Management of Skeletal Trauma in the UK,* BOA, 1992

14. R Duthie (Chairman), *Orthopaedic Services – Waiting Time for Out-Patient Appointments and In-Patient Treatment,* Report of the Working Party to the Secretary of State, DHSS, 1981

15. M Pearse and A Woolf, 'Care of elderly patients with a fractured neck of femur', *Health Trends,* Vol. 24; No. 4, 1992, pp134-5

16. E A Campling, H B Devlin, R W Hoile, J N Lunn, *The Report of the National Confidential Enquiry into Perioperative Deaths 1990*, NCEPOD, 1992

17. V J Hempsall, D R C Robertson, M J Campbell, R S Briggs, 'Orthopaedic geriatric care – is it effective? A prospective population-based comparison of outcome in fractured neck of femur', *Journal of the Royal College of Physicians of London*, Vol. 24, 1990, pp47-50

18. R Fordham, R Thompson, J Holmes, C Hodkinson, *A Cost-Benefit Study of Geriatric Orthopaedic Management of Patients with Fractured Neck of Femur*, Discussion Paper 14, University of York Centre for Health Economics, 1986

19. I Philp (ed), *Assessing Elderly People in Hospital and Community Care*, Farrand Press, 1994

20. A Squires, *Rehabilitation of the Older Patient: A Handbook for the Multidisciplinary Team*, Croom Helm, 1990

21. W Hollingworth, C Todd, M Parker, J A Roberts, R Williams, *Cost analysis of early discharge after hip fracture*, British Medical Journal, Vol. 307, 1993, pp903-6

22. Department of Health, *Discharge of Patients from Hospital*, HC(89)5 and LAC(89)7, DoH, 1989

23. Department of Health, *Hospital Discharge Workbook: A Manual on Hospital Discharge Practice*, DoH, 1994

24. Department of Health, *NHS Responsibilities for Meeting Continuing Health Care Needs*, HSG(95)8 and LAC(95)5, DoH, 1995

25. J A Mountain and C T Currie, 'Audit of hip fracture in four hospitals in Scotland', *Medical Audit News*, Vol. 5, No. 8, 1995, pp117-18

26. K-G Thorngren, *Medical Audit: Experience from Sweden*, in S P Frostick, P J Radford & W A Wallace (eds), *Medical Audit: Rationale and Practicalities*, CUP, 1993, pp365-75

Index   References are to paragraph numbers